Clinical Ethics

NOTICE

Medicine is an ever-changing science. As new research and clinical experience broaden our knowledge, changes in treatment and drug therapy are required. The authors and the publisher of this work have checked with sources believed to be reliable in their efforts to provide information that is complete and generally in accord with the standards accepted at the time of publication. However, in view of the possibility of human error or changes in medical sciences, neither the authors nor the publisher nor any other party who has been involved in the preparation or publication of this work warrants that the information contained herein is in every respect accurate or complete, and they disclaim all responsibility for any errors or omissions or for the results obtained from use of the information contained in this work. Readers are encouraged to confirm the information contained herein with other sources. For example and in particular, readers are advised to check the product information sheet included in the package of each drug they plan to administer to be certain that the information contained in this work is accurate and that changes have not been made in the recommended dose or in the contraindications for administration. This recommendation is of particular importance in connection with new or infrequently used drugs.

Fifth Edition

Clinical Ethics

A Practical Approach to Ethical Decisions in Clinical Medicine

Albert R. Jonsen, Ph.D.
Professor Emeritus of Ethics in Medicine
University of Washington School of Medicine
Seattle, Washington

Mark Siegler, M.D.
Lindy Bergman Distinguished Service Professor
  of Medicine
Director, MacLean Center for Clinical Medical Ethics
University of Chicago
Chicago, Illinois

William J. Winslade, Ph.D., J.D.
James Wade Rockwell Professor of Philosophy in Medicine
Institute for the Medical Humanities
University of Texas Medical Branch
Galveston, Texas

McGraw-Hill
Medical Publishing Division

New York • Chicago • San Francisco • Lisbon • London • Madrid • Mexico City
New Delhi • San Juan • Seoul • Singapore • Sydney • Toronto

McGraw-Hill

A Division of The *McGraw·Hill* Companies

Clinical Ethics: A Practical Approach to Ethical Decisions in
Clinical Medicine, Fifth Edition

4 5 6 7 8 9 0 DOCDOC 0 9 8 7 6 5 4

ISBN: 0-07-138763-3

This book was set in Berkley Book by ATLIS Graphics.
The editors were Isabel Nogueira and Karen Edmonson.
The production supervisor was Catherine Saggese.
The cover designer was Janice Bielawa.
The interior was designed by Mary McKeon.
R.R. Donnelley and Sons was printer and binder.

This book is printed on acid-free paper.

Library of Congress Cataloging-in-Publication Data

Jonsen, Albert R.
    Clinical ethics : a practical approach to ethical decisions in
clinical medicine / Albert R. Jonsen, Mark Siegler, William J
Winslade. —5th ed.
      p. ; cm.
    ISBN 0-07-138763-3 (softcover : alk. paper)
    1. Medical ethics.   2. Medical ethics—Case studies.   I. Siegler, Mark,
1941–   II. Winslade, William J.   III. Title.
[DNLM: 1. Ethics, Clinical.   2. Decision Making.   W 50 J81c 2002]
R724 .J66 2002
174'.2—dc21

                                                            2002023098

Contents

Introduction

THE FOUR TOPICS: CASE ANALYSIS IN CLINICAL ETHICS

Clinical ethics is a practical discipline that provides a structured approach for identifying, analyzing, and resolving ethical issues in clinical medicine. The practice of good clinical medicine requires a working knowledge about ethical issues, such as informed consent, truth telling, confidentiality, end-of-life care, pain relief, and patient rights. Medicine, even at its most technical and scientific levels, is an encounter between human beings, and the physician's work of diagnosing disease, offering advice, and providing treatment is embedded in a moral context. The willingness of physician and patient to endorse moral values, such as mutual respect, honesty, trustworthiness, compassion, and a commitment to pursue shared goals, usually ensures that significant conflicts between physician and patient rarely occur. Occasionally, physicians and patients may disagree about values or may face choices that challenge their values. It is then that ethical problems arise. Clinical ethics concerns both the ethical features that are present in every clinical encounter and the ethical problems that occasionally occur in those encounters. Clinical ethics relies on the conviction that, even when perplexity is great and emotions run high, physicians, nurses, and patients and their families can work constructively to identify, analyze, and resolve many of the ethical problems that appear in clinical medicine.

The authors have two purposes in writing this book: first, to offer an approach that facilitates thinking about the complexities of the problems that clinicians actually face and, second, to assemble concise representative opinions about typical ethical problems that occur in the practice of medicine. We do not, however, merely give answers to the ethical questions. Instead, our goal is to help clinicians understand and manage the cases they encounter in their own practices. Every clinician should recognize that ethics is an inherent aspect of good clinical medicine. Our book is intended not only for clinicians and students who provide care to patients, but also for other individuals, such as hospital administrators, hospital attorneys, members of institutional ethics committees, quality reviewers, and administrators of health plans, all of whose work requires an awareness and sensitivity to the ethical issues in clinical practice. In the complex world of modern health care, all of these persons are responsible for maintaining the ethics that lie at the heart of quality care.

Many books on health care ethics are organized around ethical principles, such as respect for autonomy, beneficence, nonmaleficence, and fairness, and cases are analyzed in the light of those principles. Other books consist of essays on particular problems, such as informed consent or forgoing life support. Our book is different. Clinical situations are complex, because they involve a wide range of medical facts, a multitude of circumstances, and a variety of values. Often, decisions must be reached quickly. The authors believe that clinicians need a straightforward method of sorting out the pertinent facts and values of any case into an orderly pattern that facilitates the discussion and resolution of ethical problems. Our book, therefore, brings together those principles and circumstances that comprise a method to facilitate the analysis of cases involving ethical issues. This technique, in our view, corresponds to the way clinicians analyze actual cases.

We suggest that every clinical case, especially those raising an ethical problem, should be analyzed by means of the following four topics: (1) medical indications, (2) patient preferences, (3) quality of life, and (4) contextual features, defined as the social, economic, legal, and administrative context in which the case occurs. Although the facts of each case can differ, these four topics are always relevant. The topics organize the various facts of the particular case and, at the same time, call attention to the ethical principles appropriate to the case. It is our intent to show readers how these four topics provide a systematic method of identifying and analyzing the ethical problems occurring in clinical medicine.

Clinicians will recall the method of case presentation that they learned at the beginning of their professional training. They were taught to "present" a patient by stating in order (1) the chief complaint, (2) history of the present illness, (3) past medical history, (4) family and social history, (5) physical findings, and (6) laboratory data. These are the topics that an experienced clinician uses to reach a diagnosis and to formulate a plan for management of the case. Although the particular details under each of these topics can differ from patient to patient, the topics themselves are constant and are always relevant to the task of arriving at a management plan. Sometimes one topic, for example, the patient's family history or the physical examination, may be particularly important or, conversely, may not be relevant to the present problem. Still, clinicians are expected to review all of the topics in every case.

Our four topics help clinicians understand how the ethical principles connect with the circumstances of the clinical case. For example, a patient comes to a physician, complaining of feeling ill. Medical indications include a clinical picture of polydipsia and polyuria, nausea, fatigue, and some mental confusion, with laboratory data indicating hyperglycemia, acidosis, and elevated plasma ketone concentrations. A diagnosis of diabetic ketoacidosis is made. Fluids and insulin are prescribed in specific doses and volumes. These clinical actions are all intended to benefit the patient. However, an ethical problem would occur if, after hearing the physician's recommendations, the patient rejects further medical attention. In these circumstances, the principle of beneficence, that is, the clinician's duty to assist the patient, and the principle of autonomy, that is, the duty to respect the patient's preferences, come into conflict with each other. As the case is described, circumstances accumulate under all four of the topics and affect the meaning and relevance of the ethical principles. It is advisable to review all four topics together to see how the principles and the circumstances together define the ethical problem in the case and suggest a resolution. Good ethical judgment consists in appreciating how ethical principles should be interpreted in the actual situation under consideration. We hope our method helps practitioners to do just that.

We divide the book into four chapters, each one devoted to one of the four topics. These four chapters define the major concepts associated with each topic, present typical cases in which the topic under discussion plays a particularly important role, and critically review the arguments commonly offered to resolve the problem. For example, the case of a Jehovah's Witness patient who refuses a blood transfusion will demonstrate how the topic of patient preferences functions in the analysis of the ethical problem presented by a patient's refusal of an indicated medical treatment. At the same time, we suggest a resolution of the case that reflects both the current opinion of medical ethicists on cases involving Jehovah's Witnesses and our own judgment. Thus, for this particular example, a reader can use this volume as a reference book, by looking up "Refusal of treatment" or "Jehovah's Witnesses" in the Locator at the back of the book and reading the several pages devoted to that issue in Chapter 2.

Those readers who use the book as a reference will find concise summaries of current opinion on the ethics of certain typical cases, such as those involving refusal of care or a diagnosis of persistent vegetative state. This information may be all that they need at the moment. However, the actual cases that clinicians encounter in practice will be a combination of unique circumstances and values. The four topics can be considered as signposts that guide the way through the complexity of real cases. Thus, using the book's four-part method as a part of clinical reasoning will serve the reader better than using it for occasional reference. The clinician will gain an appreciation of how an actual ethical case fits into the general understanding of such cases and how to reach an opinion suited to the actual case. We strongly suggest that readers read the book from beginning to end to get the full understanding of the method. We hope they will become adept at bringing the method to bear on their own clinical cases.

This book was originally written for physicians specialized in internal medicine, and it concentrated on the ethical problems encountered by those making clinical decisions for patients in their practice. In subsequent editions, the scope was broadened to adult medicine in general, and then also to pediatrics. The sections particularly relevant to pediatric ethics have the letter **P** after their numbers in the text. Also, it became obvious to the authors that many other health care providers, nurses, social workers, medical technicians, as well as chaplains and administrators, found our method useful. In this fifth edition, the original emphasis on clinical decisions made by physicians remains, but we believe that others can fit the particular concerns and values of their own professions into the topics of the book. Unfortunately, this book cannot address the ethical issues in reproductive medicine and obstetrics; the problems there involve an enigmatic third party, the fetus, and thus, they require a more complex approach than this book provides.

The method presented in this book is not only useful for clinical decision making. It also provides a simple way to determine the ethical dimensions of a patient's care. For example, the four topics might serve as the outline for a discussion between providers, patient, and family at the time of admission to an extended-care facility or to hospice care. A copy of the four topics could be given to patient and family; various questions could then be asked, and the answers recorded. This initial record could be reviewed as the patient's situation changes and as particular decisions must be made. We believe that this book, despite its use of medical language, can benefit every person who will some day be a patient, or who has family and friends who are now patients. The structured framework can guide all parties through otherwise confusing situations.

Dax's Case. We can illustrate our method by a brief summary of a case familiar to many who have studied medical ethics, namely, the case of Donald "Dax" Cowart, the burn patient who related his experience in the videotape *Please Let Me Die* and the documentary *Dax's Case*.[1]

In 1973, "Dax" Cowart, aged 25 years, was severely burned in a propane gas explosion. Rushed to the Burn Treatment Unit of Parkland Hospital in Dallas, he was found to have severe burns over 65% of his body; his face and hands suffered third-degree burns, and his eyes were severely damaged. Full-burn therapy was instituted. After an initial period during which his survival was in doubt, he was stabilized and underwent amputation of several fingers and removal of his right eye. During much of his 232-day hospitalization at Parkland, his few weeks at The Texas Institute of Rehabilitation and Research at Houston, and his subsequent 6-month stay at University of Texas Medical Branch in Galveston, he repeatedly insisted that treatment be discontinued and that he be allowed to die. Despite this demand, wound care was continued, skin grafts were performed, and nutritional and fluid support were provided. He was discharged totally blind, with minimal use of his hands, badly scarred, and dependent on others to assist in personal functions.

Discussion of the ethics involved in a case like this can begin by asking any number of questions. Did Dax have the moral or the legal right to refuse care? Was Dax competent to make a decision? Were the physicians paternalistic? What was Dax's prognosis? All these questions, and many others, are relevant and can result in vigorous debate. However, we suggest that the ethical analysis should begin by an orderly review of the four basic topics. We recommend that the same order be followed in all cases; that is, (1) medical indications, (2) patient preferences, (3) quality of life, and (4) contextual features. The use of this procedure will lay out the ethically relevant facts of the case (or show where further information is needed) before debate begins. This order of review does not constitute an order of ethical priority. The determination of relative importance of these topics will be explained in the four chapters.

Medical Indications. This topic includes the usual content of a clinical discussion: the diagnosis, prognosis, and treatment of the patient's medical problem. "Indications" refers to the diagnostic and therapeutic interventions that are appropriate to evaluate and treat the problem. Although this is the usual material covered in the presentation of any patient's clinical problems, the ethical discussion reviews the medical facts and evaluates them in the light of the fundamental ethical features of the case, such as the possibility of benefiting the patient and respecting the patient's preferences.

In Dax's case, the medical indications include the clinical facts necessary to diagnose the extent and seriousness of his burns, to make a prognosis for survival or restoration of function, and to determine the options for treatment, including the risks, benefits, and probable outcomes of each treatment modality. For example, certain prognoses are associated with burns of given severity and extent. Various forms of treatment, such as fluid replacement, skin grafting, and antibiotics are associated with certain probabilities of outcome and risk. After initial emergency treatment, Dax's prognosis for survival was approximately 20%, but the quality of life after his survival was likely to be greatly diminished by blindness, disability, and deformity. After 6 months of intensive care, his prognosis for survival improved to almost 100%. If his request to stop wound care and grafting during that first hospitalization had been respected, he would almost certainly have died. A clear view of the possible benefits of intervention is the first step in assessing the ethical aspects of a case.

Patient Preferences. In all medical treatment, the patient's preferences that are based on the patient's own values and personal assessment of benefits and burdens are ethically relevant. In every clinical case, certain questions must be asked: What does the patient want? and What are the patient's goals? The systematic review of this topic requires the following additional questions: Has the patient been provided sufficient information? Does the patient comprehend? Does the patient understand the uncertainty inherent in any medical recommendation and the range of reasonable options that exist? Is the patient consenting voluntarily? and Is the patient coerced? In some cases, an answer to these questions might be: "We don't know because the patient is incapable of formulating a preference or expressing one." If the patient is mentally incapacitated at the time a decision must be made, we must ask: Who has the authority to decide on behalf of this patient? What are the ethical and legal limits of that authority? and What is to be done if no one can be identified as surrogate?

In Dax's case, his mental capacity was questioned in the early days of his refusal of care. Had the physical and emotional shock of the accident undermined his ability to decide for himself? Initially, it was assumed that he lacked the capacity to make his own decisions, at least about refusing life-saving therapy. The doctors accepted the consent of Dax's mother in favor of treatment over his refusal of treatment. Later, when Dax was rehospitalized in the Galveston Burn Unit, a psychiatric consultation was requested, which affirmed his capacity to make decisions. Once that capacity was established, the ethical implications of his desire to refuse care became central. The following ethical questions immediately had to be considered: Should his preference be respected? Did Dax appreciate sufficiently the prospects for his rehabilitation? Are physicians obliged to pursue therapies they believe have promise over the objections of a patient? Would they be cooperating in a suicide if they assented to Dax's wishes? Any case involving the ethics of patient preferences relies on clarification of these questions.

Quality of Life. Any injury or illness threatens persons with actual or potentially reduced quality of life, manifested in the signs and symptoms of their disease. One goal of medical intervention is to restore, maintain, or improve quality of life. Thus, in all medical situations, the topic of quality of life must be considered. Many questions surround this topic: What does this phrase "quality of life" mean in general? How should it be understood in particular cases? How do persons other than the patient perceive the patient's quality of life, and of what ethical relevance are their perceptions? Above all, what is the relevance of quality of life to ethical judgment? This topic, important as it is in clinical judgment, opens the door for bias and prejudice. Still, it must be confronted in the analysis of clinical ethical problems.

In Dax's case, we note the quality of his life before the accident. He was a popular, athletic young man, just discharged from the Air Force, after serving as a fighter pilot in Vietnam. He worked in a real estate business with his father (who was also injured in the explosion and died on the way to the hospital). Before his accident, Dax's quality of life was excellent. During the course of medical care, he endured excruciating pain and profound depression. After the accident, even with the best of care, he was confronted with significant physical deficits, including notable disfigurement, blindness, and limitation of activity. During most of his hospital course, Dax had the capacity to determine what quality of life he wished for himself. However, in the early weeks of his hospitalization, he may have suffered serious deficits in mental capacity at the time critical decisions had to be made. Others would have to make quality-of-life decisions on his behalf. Was the prospect for return to a normal or even acceptable life so poor that no reasonable person would choose to live, or is any life worth living regardless of its quality? Who should make such decisions? What values should guide the decision makers? The ethical controversy occurred because Dax believed, even though his mother and physicians did not, that he had the capacity and the right to make his own quality-of-life decisions, including the right to refuse all treatment. The meaning and import of such considerations must be clarified in any clinical ethical analysis.

Contextual Features. Preferences and quality of life bring out the most common features of the medical encounter. However, every medical case is embedded in a larger context of persons, institutions, and financial and social arrangements. The possibilities and the constraints of that context influence patient care, positively or negatively. At the same time, the context itself is affected by the decisions made by or about the patient: these decisions may have psychological, emotional, financial, legal, scientific, educational, or religious impact on others. In every case, the relevance of the contextual features must be determined and assessed. These contextual features may be crucially important to the understanding and resolution of the case.

In Dax's case, several of these contextual features were significant. Dax's mother was opposed to termination of his medical care for religious reasons. The legal implications of honoring Dax's demand were unclear at the time. The costs of 16 months of intensive burn therapy were substantial. Dax's refusal to cooperate with treatment may have influenced the attitudes of physicians and nurses toward him. These and other contextual factors must be made explicit and assessed for their relevance.

Rules and Principles. These four topics are relevant to any clinical case, whatever the actual circumstances. They serve as a useful organizing device for teaching and discussion. Some clinicians have even found them useful for organizing a plan for patient management. A review of these topics can also help to move the discussion of an ethical problem toward a resolution. Any serious discussion of an ethical problem must go beyond merely talking about it in an orderly way: it must push through to a reasonable and practical resolution. Ethical problems, no less than medical problems, cannot be left hanging. Thus, after presenting a case, the task of seeking a resolution must begin.

The discussion of each topic includes certain standards of behavior that are ethically appropriate to the topic. These can be called ethical principles or ethical rules. For example, one version of the principle of beneficence states, "There is an obligation to assist others in the furthering of their legitimate interests." The ethical rule, "Physicians have a duty to treat patients, even at risk to themselves," is a specific expression of that broad principle, suited to a particular sphere of professional activity, namely, medical care. The topic of medical indications, in addition to the clinical data that must be discussed, includes the additional questions, "How much can we do to help this patient?" and "What risks of adverse effects can be tolerated in the attempt to treat the patient?" Answers to these questions, arising so naturally in the discussion of medical indications, can be guided by familiar historical rules of medical ethics such as, "Be of benefit and do no harm" or "Risks should be balanced by benefits." Rules such as these reflect in a specific way the broad principle that the philosophers have named beneficence. Similarly, the topic of patient preferences contains rules that instruct clinicians to tell patients the truth, to respect their deliberate preferences, and to honor their values. Rules such as these fall under the general scope of the principles of autonomy and respect for persons.

Our method of analysis begins, not with the principles and rules, as do many other ethics treatises, but with the factual features of the case. We refer to principles and rules as they become relevant to the discussion of the topics. In this way, abstract discussion of principles is avoided, as is also the tendency to think of only one principle, such as autonomy or beneficence, as the sole guide in the case. Ethical rules and principles are best appreciated in the specific context of the actual circumstances of a case. For example, a key issue in Dax's case is the autonomy of the patient. However, the significance of autonomy in Dax's case is derived not simply from the principle that requires we respect it, but from the confluence of considerations about preferences, medical indications for treatment, quality of life, decisional capacity, and the role of his mother, the doctors, the lawyers, and the hospitals. Only when all these are seen and evaluated in relation to each other will the meaning of the principle of autonomy be appreciated in this case.

Research in Medical Ethics. Competence in clinical ethics depends not only on the ability to use a sound method for analysis, but also on a familiarity with the literature of medical ethics. Some readers will seek further elaboration of the issues dealt with so briefly in this book. We rarely cite articles (except those that we quote), because the literature in bioethics is extensive and in constant evolution. Instead, we refer, when useful, to the most widely used general text in bioethics, Beauchamp and Childress, *Principles of Biomedical Ethics*.[2] We also reference the Special Issues and Special Sections of three principal American journals in bioethics, *Hastings Center Report*,[3] *Journal of Clinical Ethics*,[4] and *Cambridge Quarterly of Healthcare Ethics*.[5] These special issues and sections provide broad views of particular issues with bibliographies of the current literature. Readers seeking the most current articles may search in the annual publication *The Bibliography of Bioethics*.[6] This source is available on-line as Bioethicsline, through the National Library of Medicine's MEDLARS. There are also many useful Web sites, such as those of the Clinical Ethics Center of the National Institutes of Health, http://www.nih.gov/sigs/bioethics.

Four Cases. Four clinical cases will reappear throughout this book as our major examples. The patients in these cases are given the names Mr. Cure, Ms. Care, Ms. Comfort, and Mr. Cope. These fictional names are chosen to suggest certain prominent features of their medical condition. Mr. Cure suffers from bacterial meningitis, a serious but curable acute condition. Ms. Comfort has breast cancer that has metastasized, for which there is a low probability of cure even under a regimen of intensive intervention. Ms. Care has multiple sclerosis, a disease that cannot be cured but whose inexorable deterioration can be managed by continual care. Mr. Cope has a chronic condition, insulin-dependent diabetes, that requires certain medical assistance but depends heavily on the patient's active involvement in his own care. Details of these cases will occasionally be changed to illustrate various points as the text proceeds. Many other shorter case examples will appear in which the patients will be designated by initials.

Case I. Mr. Cure, a 24-year-old man, has been brought to the emergency room by a friend. Previously in good health, he is complaining of severe headache and a stiff neck. The results of the physical examination and laboratory studies, including spinal fluid examination, suggest a diagnosis of pneumococcal pneumonia and pneumococcal meningitis.

Case II. Mr. Cope is a 42-year-old man with insulin-dependent diabetes. His diabetes was first diagnosed at age 18. He complied with an insulin and dietary regimen quite faithfully. Still, he experienced frequent episodes of ketoacidosis and hypoglycemia, which necessitated repeated hospitalizations and emergency room care. For the last few years, his diabetes has been controlled, and he required hospitalization only once for ketoacidosis associated with acute pyelonephritis. Twenty-one years after the onset of diabetes, he appears to have no functional impairment from his disease. However, fundoscopic examination reveals a moderate number of microaneurysms and urinalysis shows persistent proteinuria. He has no neurologic symptoms or abnormal physical findings.

Case III. Mrs. Care, a 44-year-old married woman with two children, was diagnosed with multiple sclerosis (MS) 15 years ago. Over the past 12 years, the patient has experienced progressive deterioration. She developed severe spasticity in both legs, requiring canes, then a walker, and finally full use of a wheelchair. She is now blind in one eye, with markedly decreased vision in the other. For the past 2 years, she has required an indwelling Foley catheter because of an atonic bladder. In the last year, she has become profoundly depressed, is uncommunicative even with close family, and refuses to rise from bed.

Case IV. Ms. Comfort is a 58-year-old woman. She has had a mammogram yearly for the past 6 years. Eight months after her last mammogram, she noted a rapidly enlarging right breast mass. She was seen by her primary care physician and referred to a surgeon who performed a breast biopsy that confirmed the presence of an infiltrating ductal adenocarcinoma. She underwent a modified radical mastectomy with reconstruction. Dissected nodes revealed metastatic disease. She received a course of chemotherapy and radiation.

On page 12, a chart depicts the four topics in quadrants. This chart can serve as a convenient way to record the facts of a case in an orderly way. However, it has a much more important purpose as a guide for ethical deliberation about a case. The many facts do not remain isolated in their respective quadrants. Rather, once they are displayed, the ethical task begins: to evaluate the facts in relation to each other and in light of the principles. In some cases, once the facts are clear, it also becomes clear that the issue is easily resolved: confusion about the facts or failures in communication may have obscured the obvious priority of one or another principle. In other cases, reflective balancing of the principles is required, so as to reveal which principle should take priority. Finally, there are cases where the facts and the principles may be clear, but a genuine ethical dilemma may remain. We are aware that there are such dilemmas in clinical medicine, but we are convinced that many ethical problems can be reasonably resolved. When value conflicts are encountered, reasonable persons should make choices only after careful, honest consideration of the ethical aspects and the facts of the situation. We hope that this book will assist persons in doing just that.

REFERENCES

1. Kliever LD, ed. *Dax's Case. Essays in Medical Ethics and Human Meaning.* Dallas: Southern Methodist University Press, 1989.

2. Beauchamp TL, Childress JF. *Principles of Biomedical Ethics.* 4th ed. New York: Oxford University Press, 1994.

3. *Hastings Center Report.* The Hastings Center, Garrison, New York, 10524-5555. Email: mail@thehastingscenter.org.

4. *Journal of Clinical Ethics.* 17100 Cole Road, Hagerstown, MD 21740. www.clinicalethics.com.

5. *Cambridge Quarterly of Healthcare Ethics.* 40 West 20th Street, New York, NY 10011-4211. www.journals.cup.org.

6. Walters L, Kahn TJ, eds. *Bibliography of Bioethics.* Washington, DC: Georgetown University. Published annually. Online as BIOETHICSLINE, National Library of Medicine, MEDLARS.

■ MEDICAL INDICATIONS

The Principles of Beneficence and
Nonmaleficence

1. What is the patient's medical problem?
   history? diagnosis? prognosis?
2. Is the problem acute? chronic? critical?
   emergent? reversible?
3. What are the goals of treatment?
4. What are the probabilities of success?
5. What are the plans in case of
   therapeutic failure?
6. In sum, how can this patient be
   benefited by medical and nursing care,
   and how can harm be avoided?

■ PATIENT PREFERENCES

The Principle of Respect for Autonomy

1. Is the patient mentally capable and
   legally competent? Is there evidence of
   incapacity?
2. If competent, what is the patient
   stating about preferences for treatment?
3. Has the patient been informed of
   benefits and risks, understood
   this information, and given consent?
4. If incapacitated, who is the appropriate
   surrogate? Is the surrogate using appropriate standards for decision making?
5. Has the patient expressed prior
   preferences, e.g., Advance Directives?
6. Is the patient unwilling or unable to
   cooperate with medical treatment?
   If so, why?
7. In sum, is the patient's right to choose
   being respected to the extent possible
   in ethics and law?

■ QUALITY OF LIFE

The Principles of Beneficence and
Nonmaleficence and Respect for
Autonomy

1. What are the prospects, with or
   without treatment, for a return to
   normal life?
2. What physical, mental, and social
   deficits is the patient likely to
   experience if treatment succeeds?
3. Are there biases that might prejudice
   the provider's evaluation of the patient's
   quality of life?
4. Is the patient's present or future condition such that his or her continued life
   might be judged undesirable?
5. Is there any plan and rationale to forgo
   treatment?
6. Are there plans for comfort and
   palliative care?

■ CONTEXTUAL FEATURES

The Principles of Loyalty and Fairness

1. Are there family issues that might
   influence treatment decisions?
2. Are there provider (physicians and
   nurses) issues that might influence
   treatment decisions?
3. Are there financial and economic
   factors?
4. Are there religious or cultural factors?
5. Are there limits on confidentiality?
6. Are there problems of allocation of
   resources?
7. How does the law affect treatment
   decisions?
8. Is clinical research or teaching involved?
9. Is there any conflict of interest on the
   part of the providers or the institution?

Chapter 1

1.0 ▪ ▪ ▪ ▪ ▪ ▪ ▪ ▪ ▪ ▪ ▪ ▪

Indications for Medical Intervention

This chapter treats the first topic relevant to any ethical problem in clinical medicine, namely, the indications for or against medical intervention. These indications are the facts about the patient's health that prompt the diagnostic and therapeutic activities that comprise modern medical care. They imply the overall goals of medicine: prevention, cure, and care of illness and injury. In most cases, treatment decisions that are based on medical indications are straightforward and present no obvious ethical problems. For example, a patient complains of frequent urination accompanied by a burning sensation; the physician suspects a urinary tract infection, obtains a confirmatory culture, and prescribes an antibiotic. The physician explains to the patient the nature of the condition and the reason for prescribing the medication. The patient obtains the prescription, takes the medication, and is cured of the infection. This case exemplifies clinical ethics, not because it shows an ethical problem, but because the treatment goals and ethical values are shared by both the physician and the patient. Medical indications are clear enough for the physician to make a diagnosis and prescribe an effective therapy to benefit the patient. The patient's preferences coincide with the physician's recommendations, and the patient's quality of life, presently rendered unpleasant by the infection, is improved. Insurance pays the bill, medications are available, and no other complications occur. The ethical principles of respect for autonomy, beneficence, and nonmaleficence and loyalty are satisfied.

In some cases, however, ethical problems do appear. In the previous case, ethical problems would appear if the patient stated that he did not believe in antibiotics, or if the urinary tract infection developed in the last days of a terminal illness, or if the infection was clearly associated with a sexually transmitted disease where sexual partners might be endangered, or if the patient could not pay for the care. Sometimes, these problems can be readily resolved; at other times, they can become major obstacles in the management of the case. The patient's medical status is crucial to the understanding of any ethical problem that might appear in the case. Medical status includes the nature of the disease, its prognosis, whether it is treated or not, treatment alternatives, and, above all, the goals of the intervention.

In this chapter, we define medical indications and discuss some features of clinical medicine relating to medical indications, including the goals and benefits of medicine, the patient-physician relationship and professionalism, clinical judgment and uncertainty, evidence-based medicine, and medical error. We then consider four ethical issues that depend heavily on the indications for or against medical interventions: (1) medical futility, (2) cardiopulmonary resuscitation and do-not-resuscitate orders, (3) good care of the dying patient, and (4) the definition of death.

1.0.1 Definition of Medical Indications

Every discussion of an ethical problem in clinical medicine should begin with a statement of the medical facts. This statement should follow the pattern familiar to medical students and physicians when they present a patient for clinical purposes: presenting complaint, history, results of physical examination, laboratory and other diagnostic studies, presumptive diagnosis, prognosis, and management plan. These data indicate the appropriate approach to the treatment of the patient. In the usual clinical presentation, this review of indications for medical intervention leads to the formulation of recommendations to the patient for further diagnostic studies and treatment regimens.

Case. Mr. Cure, a 24-year-old white graduate student, has been brought to the emergency room by a friend. Previously in good health, he is complaining of a severe headache and stiff neck. Physical examination shows a somnolent patient without focal neurologic signs but with a temperature of 39.5 °C and nuchal rigidity. An examination of spinal fluid reveals cloudy fluid with a white count of 2,000; a Gram's stain of the fluid shows many gram-positive diplococci. A diagnosis of bacterial meningitis is reached.

In this case, the medical indications are based on the diagnosis of bacterial meningitis for which a specific therapy, namely, administration of antibiotics, is appropriate. Nothing yet suggests that this case poses any ethical problem. However, in Chapter 2, we shall encounter an ethical problem in this case: Mr. Cure will refuse therapy. That refusal will cause consternation among the physicians and the nurses caring for him; it will also raise a genuine ethical problem about the duty of physicians to benefit the patient versus the autonomy of the patient. Rather than plunging into what seems to be the ethical problem, namely, the patient's refusal, any proper analysis of the case must begin with a clear exposition of the medical indications. In other words, the analysis should begin not with the question "Does a patient have the right to refuse treatment of a life-threatening condition?" but with answers to the questions, "What is the diagnosis?" "What are the medical indications for treatment?" and "Are there any reasonable alternatives for treating this clinical problem?"

1.0.2 The Goals and Benefits of Medicine

The practice of medicine consists of a relationship between a patient and a physician. The goals and benefits of medicine are optimal in relationships where physicians and other health professionals demonstrate a professionalism that includes honesty and integrity, respect for patients, a commitment to patients' welfare, a compassionate regard for patients, and a dedication to maintaining competency in knowledge and technical skills. The physician's central responsibility is to use that medical competence to respond to the patient's need for help. The physician makes a diagnosis and recommends a course of action. That course of action will have some or all of the following goals:

1. Promotion of health and prevention of disease
2. Relief of symptoms, pain, and suffering
3. Cure of disease
4. Prevention of untimely death
5. Improvement of functional status or maintenance of compromised status
6. Education and counseling of patients regarding their condition and prognosis
7. Avoidance of harm to the patient in the course of care

The achievement of these goals is the benefit of medicine. Frequently, all or most of these can be achieved simultaneously. In Mr. Cure's case, the administration of antibiotics should relieve symptoms and cure the disease, thereby preventing Mr. Cure's death and restoring his health. Sometimes it is difficult to accomplish all desirable goals for several reasons: (1) a conflict between diverse goals, (2) the difficulty of attaining a positive goal without doing harm, and (3) a lack of clarity about the goals.

Special Supplement: The Goals of Medicine: Setting New Priorities. *Hastings Cent Rep* 1996;26(suppl)(6):1–27.

EXAMPLES. (a) A middle-aged man has repeated blood pressures of 175/110, which have not improved with behavioral changes in diet, weight control, and smoking cessation. He has tried several kinds of antihypertensive drugs, but each class of drugs has caused side effects, such as impotence, constipation, and fatigue. He is discouraged. His physician explains that control of blood pressure will reduce risk of heart attack and stroke. The patient considers whether the future statistical benefit of reducing risks is worth the present side effects of drug treatment.

(b) Combined antiretroviral therapy clearly delays the progression of HIV infection, often improves quality of life, and prolongs survival. The degree of long-term benefit remains uncertain. These drugs may have certain side effects, particularly, nausea, diarrhea, and kidney stones. They require patients to take up to 14 tablets per day in accordance with a rigorous schedule and cost approximately $12,000 per year. The use of combination therapy for preventive purposes poses a difficult trade-off between risks and benefits. The goal of delaying symptoms may be compromised by the goal of avoiding harm: in this case, the serious side effects, the burden of the drug regimen, the cost of the drugs, and the uncertain long-term benefits of such a regimen.

1.0.3 The Ethical Principles of Beneficence and Nonmaleficence

The work of caring for patients in such a way as to maximize benefit and to avoid harm rests on two ethical principles, usually called **beneficence** and **nonmaleficence**. The presence of medical indications raises the question, "How can a medical intervention help this patient?" This question reflects one of the central ethical maxims of medical practice, stated in the Hippocratic oath: "I will use treatment to help the sick according to my ability and judgment but never with a view to injury and wrongdoing." Another Hippocratic writing states, "As to diseases make a habit of two things: to help or at least to do no harm" (Epidemics I, xi). These maxims exemplify the ethical principles of beneficence, the duty to assist persons in need, and its converse, nonmaleficence, the duty to refrain from causing harm. The ethical responsibilities of physicians are closely tied to their ability to fulfill the goals of medicine in conjunction with the patients' preferences about the goals of their lives. The principles of beneficence and nonmaleficence require the physician to evaluate the potential benefits of any proposed intervention in relation to its risks, to make a recommendation to the patient, and to solicit the patient's preferences about whether to undergo the treatment.

Pellegrino ED, Thomasma D. *For the Patient's Benefit: The Restoration of Beneficence in Health Care.* New York: Oxford University Press; 1988;113–214.

1.0.4 Clinical Judgment and Clinical Uncertainty

When the goals of the intervention are unclear, or when previously clear goals become obscure, ethical questions are asked, such as "What are we accomplishing?" "Is the expected outcome worth the effort?" and "Do the benefits justify the risks?" Ethical reflection must begin with a realistic evaluation of the goals of intervention. The results of this evaluation must form the basis for the physician's opinion about the possible courses of action and must be presented to the patient or the patient's surrogate. The process by which a physician reaches a clinical judgment requires the ability to gather data, discern relevant differences, discard extraneous facts, reason probabilistically about the possible courses of action, and recommend the course that seems best. In clinical medicine, each of these steps is attended with some uncertainty.

Clinical medicine was described by Dr. William Osler as "a science of uncertainty and an art of probability." The central task of clinicians is to reduce uncertainty by using data-gathering skills, medical knowledge, and clinical reasoning to reach a diagnosis and propose a plan of care that meets the patient's needs. The process by which discerning clinicians, faced with clinical uncertainty, attempt to make consistently good decisions is called **clinical judgment.** In conjunction with the personal side of medicine—empathy, respect for persons, effective communication skills, and commitment to the patient's interests—clinical judgment constitutes the "art of medicine." This art was long believed to be an intuitive process, too complex to be subjected to analysis or scientific study. In recent years, a challenge to the traditional view about clinical judgment has come from clinical epidemiology and evidence-based medicine. These approaches assert that clinical medicine is a science and that the disciplines of clinical biostatistics, clinical epidemiology, and decision analysis can be used to evaluate the quality of both physicians' recommendations and patients' outcomes.

Feinstein AR. *Clinical Judgment.* New York: Kreiger; 1974.

Evidence-based medicine aims at the reduction of uncertainty. Proponents of evidence-based medicine suggest that decisions about therapy should be based on solid evidence derived from well-conducted, randomized controlled trials or cohort studies and, absent such evidence, on the less convincing evidence from case-controlled studies and expert clinical opinion. Evidence should show that a treatment is effective and that its prospective benefits outweigh its harms. "Practice guidelines," which prompt a physician's reasoning through a clinical problem, are developed on the basis of such evidence. Clinical guidelines should certainly not be construed as recipes for treatment, because clinical studies come to statistical conclusions and do not reflect the actual patient who is seen by the physician. Although the "uncertainty" and "probability" of which Osler spoke remain, clinical science aims to reduce these effects through the prudent use of evidence-based medicine.

A fundamental change in the relationship between patients and physicians has been a gradual shift, during the past few decades, in decisional authority from the physician to the patient. Advocates of evidence-based medicine agree that, even when the physician's recommendation is based on sound evidence, the patient is the best decision maker, because only the patient can assess the risks, benefits, goals, and costs of treatment in the face of the clinical uncertainty that will always be present in medicine. We discuss the role of patient preferences in Chapter 2.

Thus, the physician makes a recommendation after judicious reflection on the available facts and his or her interpretation on the basis of the best available data, concluding that a particular course of action best suits both the patient's medical needs and personal goals and preferences. Physicians also recognize that judgments about medical indications are not wholly derived from facts. Their judgments are colored by personal values in many respects, such as an activist or conservative attitude about intervention, peer esteem, career advancement, or a compassionate or skeptical view of the human condition. Emotions that a physician may be reluctant to admit may bias outwardly "objective" judgments: anxiety regarding death and disability, dislike of certain types of persons or lifestyles, racial prejudices, gender bias, repugnance for aged or retarded persons, or a desire for economic profit. Physicians should be aware of any attitudes that may distort their clinical reasoning.

1.0.5 Medical Error

Physicians not only work under uncertainty; they also may make mistakes. A recent study on medical error estimated that between 44,000 and 98,000 Americans die each year as a result of medical errors, more than die of vehicular accidents or breast cancer or AIDS. In this report, safety was defined as freedom from accidental injury; error was defined as the failure of a planned action to be completed as intended, or as the use of a wrong plan to achieve an aim. The report highlighted the personal and financial costs of error and noted that some errors were due to incompetence or errors of judgment by competent physicians. Other errors were caused by system failures that often went unrecognized and uncorrected. When medical error occurs as a result of incompetence or remediable ignorance, it constitutes a serious breach of the physician's clinical and ethical responsibility. Medical error produces ethical problems related to truth telling, which will be discussed in Chapter 2. Systemic error is an issue of organizational ethics, treated in Chapter 4.

Institute of Medicine. *To Err Is Human: Building a Safer Health System.* Washington, DC: National Academy Press; 1999.

Sharpe VA, Faden AI. *Medical Harm: Historical, Conceptual and Ethical Dimensions of Iatrogenic Illness.* New York: Cambridge University Press; 1998.

Special Issue on Medical Error. *J Clin Ethics* 1997;8(4):323–358.

1.0.6 Important Distinctions

To understand the clinical situation of the patient, certain disease conditions must be distinguished to appreciate the nature of disease, treatment, and clinical outcome. The ethical aspects of the case will often depend on a clear perception of these different conditions.

The Disease: Disease conditions may be (a) *acute* (having rapid onset, severe symptoms, and short course) or *chronic* (with a persistent, usually progressive course over a long period); (b) *critical* or *emergent* (causing immediate, serious, and irreversible functional disabilities, including death, unless treatment is immediately applied) or *noncritical* or *nonemergent* (slowly progressive, even when serious, but not immediately life-threatening); (c) *reversible* (course can be altered by definitive, effective therapy) or *irreversible* (symptoms or acute crises can be managed, but course progresses inevitably toward death).

The Treatment: Modalities of intervention may be (a) *curative* (a treatment, such as a course of antibiotics for simple infection or surgical operation for hernia, will definitively correct the disease condition) or *supportive* (relieving symptoms or reducing deterioration during the entire course of a chronic, irreversible disease, such as diabetes); (b) *burdensome* (causing adverse effects that are painful, disfiguring, or disabling, such as some cancer chemotherapy) or *nonburdensome* (unlikely to have perceptible or serious side effects, such as moderate exercise for prevention of mild obesity or antibiotic treatment of acute bladder infection).

The goals of intervention differ in relation to these conditions. One common ethical problem occurs when a person with a chronic, nonemergent, irreversible disease (such as multiple sclerosis) is seen with an acute, emergent, and reversible problem (such as a myocardial infarction). The goals of intervention relevant to the latter condition must be evaluated in light of the goals proper to the former. For example, a definitive treatment, such as a successful cardiopulmonary resuscitation in a terminally ill cancer patient, may do nothing more than prolong a painful dying episode. Returning to the case of Mr. Cure, the patient with meningitis (Section 1.0.1), the goals of medical intervention seem obvious. The patient has pneumococcal meningitis, an acute, critical, and reversible medical problem that can be treated easily with a course of antibiotics. However, given certain changes in the medical facts of the case, the goals of intervention may change. For example, if Mr. Cure were known to be terminally ill because of metastatic cancer, the goal of reversing an acute, lethal condition would be less obvious.

1.0 P Medical Indications and Goals in Pediatrics

The description and resolution of ethical problems in pediatrics proceeds in the same fashion as in adult medicine. First, the medical indications for diagnostic and therapeutic interventions with respect to the patient's physical condition should be reviewed. These indications must reflect the goals of medical practice and the responsibilities of pediatricians. In general, the responsibilities of pediatricians are the same as those of other physicians: to benefit the patient and to refrain from harm. The goals of medical intervention are the same, whether the patient is adult or infant: restoration of health, relief of symptoms, restoration of impaired function, saving life, and preventing untimely death. A particularly important pediatric goal is the prevention of disease and injury through the education of parents. In pediatric medicine, the exercise of these responsibilities has some special features as follows:

1. Infants at the beginning of life have no capacity for preferences; young children are often too immature to formulate preferences.
2. Parents or guardians have the moral and legal responsibility to act in the child's best interest. When questions arise about conflicts of interest or the wisdom of the parents' or guardians' choices, the scope of their authority may require legal limitation.
3. The interests of the patient may be affected by the family situation, such as the interest of siblings, economic factors, or religious beliefs. Family values, not only individual preferences, shape the interpretation of benefits for the child.
4. As children mature, their preferences become increasingly important in reaching decisions about appropriate treatment.

These features of pediatric medicine may modify the exercise of the basic responsibilities of physicians. In particular, the duty to respect the choices of autonomous persons differs significantly when the person with whom the physician communicates is a parent or guardian rather than the patient. Practitioners in pediatric specialties may be held to a more stringent duty to formulate an independent judgment of what course would be in the patient's best interest and to test and even to challenge proxy decisions against this standard.

Special Issue on Ethics in Pediatrics. *J Clin Ethics* 2000;11(2):145–150.

1.1 INAPPROPRIATE INTERVENTIONS

Modern medicine has available innumerable interventions, from advice to drugs to surgery. Each of these interventions must be clearly related to the clinical situation and to the goals of medicine. The competent clinician must judge which of these interventions is appropriate for the case at hand. Interventions may be inappropriate for a variety of reasons. First, the intervention may have no scientifically demonstrated effect on the disease to be treated and yet be erroneously selected by the clinician or desired by the patient. An example of such an intervention would be high-dose chemotherapy followed by bone marrow transplantation for widely metastatic breast cancer. Second, an intervention known to be efficacious in general may not have the usual effect in some patients because of individual differences in constitution or in the disease. An example of this type of intervention would be a patient who is administered a cholesterol-lowering statin drug and subsequently experiences an acute myopathy, a rare but known serious complication. Third, an appropriate intervention at one time in the patient's course may cease to be appropriate at a later time. An example of this would be ventilatory support applied at a patient's admission for cardiac arrest but no longer indicated when the patient suffers multisystem organ failure unresponsive to intensive care.

This last situation occurs when a patient is so seriously ill or injured that sound clinical judgment would suggest that the goals of restoration of health and function are unattainable and, thus, certain medical interventions are not indicated or should be limited. These cases present themselves in several ways: the moribund patient, the terminal patient, and the "hopelessly ill" patient. A single case, that of Mrs. Care, with some clinical variations, can illustrate these three situations.

Case. Mrs. Care, a 48-year-old married woman with two children, was diagnosed as having multiple sclerosis (MS) 15 years ago. Her initial symptoms consisted of numbness and weakness of her right leg and decreased visual acuity in the left eye. These signs resolved, but 2 years later, she developed spasticity and weakness in her left leg. During the past 12 years, the patient has experienced progressive deterioration. She developed severe spasticity in both legs, requiring a cane, then a walker, and finally, full use of a wheelchair. She is now blind in one eye, with markedly decreased vision in the other. She has been given several multiple sclerosis drugs but has failed to show any significant response. Since developing an atonic bladder 5 years ago, she has required an indwelling Foley catheter and has developed several urinary tract infections. She has been to the hospital several times for management of pyelonephritis and urosepsis. She has difficulty controlling oral secretions and has been hospitalized twice in the last year for aspiration pneumonia. In the course of the last year, she has become profoundly depressed, is uncommunicative even with close family, and refuses to leave her bed. During the entire course of her illness, she has refused to discuss the issue of terminal care, saying she found such discussion depressing and discouraging.

1.1.1 The Moribund Patient

The word "moribund" literally means "about to die." Certain clinical conditions indicate definitively that the patient's organ systems are disintegrating rapidly and irreversibly. Death can be expected within hours. In this situation, indications for medical intervention change significantly.

Case. Mrs. Care, in the advanced stages of MS, suffers from deep decubitus ulcers and osteomyelitis, neither of which has responded to treatment efforts, including skin grafts. During the past month, the patient has been admitted 3 times to the ICU with aspiration pneumonia and has required mechanical ventilation. She is admitted again, requiring ventilation and, after 4 days, becomes septic. On the next day, she is noted to have increasingly stiff lungs and poor oxygenation. In several hours, her BP is 60/40, is decreasing, and is unresponsive to pressors and volume. She is anuric and her arterial pH is 6.92. A house officer asks whether ventilation and pressors should be discontinued.

COMMENT. Medical intervention at this point is sometimes called futile, that is, offering no therapeutic benefit to the patient. In this case, the word "futile" is used in its least controversial way, that is, as "physiologic futility," a condition in which physical deterioration has progressed to the point where no known intervention can restore function. This patient now has adult respiratory disease syndrome (ARDS) in which acute lung injury progresses relentlessly to fibrosis, and the lungs permanently lose the capability for gas exchange. Mechanical support will not reverse this situation. Thus, because the patient does not and cannot respond

physiologically to treatment, any efforts will be "physiologically futile."
The concept of futility is more fully discussed at Section 1.1.3.

RECOMMENDATION. Mrs. Care is now moribund. Her death will take place
within hours. Ventilation and vasopressor are no longer indicated.
Physiologic futility is an ethical reason for the physician to recommend
withdrawing all interventions, with the exception of those that provide
comfort. If the patient's family requests continued treatment, see the discussion in Chapter 2.

1.1.2 The Terminal Patient

There is no standard clinical definition of "terminal." The word is often
loosely used to refer to the prognosis of any patient with a lethal disease.
Under Medicare and Medicaid eligibility rules, reimbursement for hospice care defines terminal as having 6 months or less to live. This is an administrative rather than a clinical definition of terminal. "Terminal"
should be applied only to those patients who experienced clinicians expect will die from a specified disease, despite appropriate treatment, in a
relatively short period, measured in days, weeks, or several months at
most. Diagnosis of a terminal condition should be made cautiously but realistically and should be based on medical evidence and clinical judgment. The benefits of accurate prognostication include informing patients
about their situation, permitting advance care planning, and allowing
physicians and patients to reach good clinical decisions. More than a few
studies have shown that even experienced clinicians often fail to make
prognoses that are verified in fact. Some physicians are overly pessimistic,
but one major study shows that even more clinicians are inappropriately
optimistic and fail to inform patients of their imminent death.

Christakis N. *Death Foretold: Prophecy and Prognosis in Medical Care.* Chicago:
University of Chicago Press; 1999.

Case. Mrs. Care is living at home. She requires assistance in all activities
of daily life and is confined to bed. She has become confused and disoriented. She begins to experience breathing difficulties. She is brought
to the emergency department. She is now unresponsive, and has a high
fever and labored, shallow respirations. A chest radiograph reveals diffuse haziness suggestive of adult respiratory distress syndrome; arterial
blood gases show a P_{O_2} of 35, P_{CO_2} of 85, and pH of 7.02. Cardiac studies demonstrate an acute anteroseptal myocardial infarction. Neurologic
and pulmonary consultants agree that she has primary neuromuscular
respiratory insufficiency. Should Mrs. Care be intubated and admitted to
the intensive care unit?

COMMENT. This acute episode is clearly life-threatening. Various interventions might delay Mrs. Care's demise. A respirator may improve gas exchange and support perfusion of organ systems; fibrinolytic therapy or angioplasty plus stenting might limit the evolving infarct. These interventions aim at two of the goals of medicine: support of compromised function and prolongation of life. Given the presence of progressive and irreversible disease in its final stages and radical damage to multiple organ systems, none of medicine's other important goals can be achieved. The patient will certainly never be restored to health; pain and symptoms will not be alleviated; and compromised functions will not be restored but sustained temporarily by mechanical means. The following reflections are relevant:

(a) Mrs. Care has expressed no preferences about the course of her care, and nothing is known from other sources about her preferences. Thus, personal preferences, usually so important in these decisions, are not relevant. The objective data about survival and sound clinical discretion about the probabilities of improvement are determinative in the recommendation to forgo further treatment.

(b) Considering the complexities of this patient's situation, the probabilities of her recovery to health, or even to her limited condition before this hospitalization approach zero. Although her pneumonia and myocardial infarction might be successfully treated, the neuromuscular cause of the pneumonia, resulting from her MS, cannot be reversed. Mrs. Care has entered the terminal phase of her illness, and her death is imminent, even though she is not yet moribund. Her survival, even under the best of circumstances, will probably be no more than several weeks. Thus, medical interventions will not effect any improvement, except, perhaps, a temporary relief of pneumonia, and will not promote any of the goals of medicine, with the possible exception of brief prolongation of life in its terminal stage.

(c) From the viewpoint of medical indications, physicians have no obligation to prolong life independent of their obligation to fulfill at least some of the other goals of medicine. The tradition of medical ethics has taken this position. In the Hippocratic writing entitled *The Art*, the physician is advised to "assuage the suffering of the sick, lessen the violence of their diseases and refuse to treat those who are overmastered by their diseases, recognizing that in such cases medicine is powerless." This wise advice prevailed until recently, and we believe it should still be honored. Regrettably, contemporary practice too often pursues a prolongation of organic life that, in the absence of any other human capacities, provides no benefit to the patient. This is a failure to recognize, or a refusal to admit that, in such cases, medicine can only postpone, not prevent, death.

(d) Objective information that provides prognostic criteria may be useful in determining whether a particular type of intervention will be efficacious. Such objective information may include the patient's diagnosis, physiologic condition, functional status, and comorbidities, together with the patient's estimated likelihood of recovery. One approach to developing these data for patients admitted to the ICU is the Acute Physiological and Chronic Health Evaluation (APACHE). This system combines an acute physiologic score, the Glasgow Coma Score, age, and a chronic disease score to estimate a patient's risk of dying during an ICU admission. Such an analysis done for this patient with pneumonia, ARDS, and acute MI would show that the probability of her surviving this ICU admission is extremely low. Even though probability is not equivalent to certainty, it is in this instance, as everywhere else in medicine, a sound basis for clinical judgment. This situation can be described as "probabilistic futility."

Knaus WA, Wagner DP, Draper EA, et al. APACHE III Prognostic System. Risk prediction of hospital mortality for critically ill, hospitalized adults. *Chest* 1991;100:1619–1636.

1.1.3 Medical Futility

Medical interventions are sometimes described as "futile." This term has many meanings, and its use in clinical ethics is hotly debated. *The Oxford English Dictionary* defines it as "incapable of producing any result, failing utterly of the desired end through intrinsic defect." In Section 1.1.1 we have seen the term "futility" refer to "physiologic futility," that is, an utter impossibility that the desired physiologic response (in that case, the restored capability for air exchange) can be effected by any intervention. In the clinical situation, futility more often designates an effort to provide a benefit to a patient, which reason and experience suggest is highly likely to fail and whose rare exceptions cannot be systematically produced. Here the judgment of futility is probabilistic, and its accuracy depends on empirical data drawn from clinical trials and from clinical experience. This is the so-called quantitative futility, which we prefer to call "probabilistic futility." Because clinical studies relative to this situation are rare, and experience is so varied, clinicians have widely different judgments: physicians' judgments that various procedures should be called futile range from 0 to 50%, clustering about 10%. Finally, futility has a qualitative meaning: the judgment that the goal that might be attained is not worthwhile. All uses of the term "futility" represent value judgments, but the qualitative meaning is most obviously based on the preferences of clinicians and patients. Some ethicists deny the utility of the concept of futility, because of its confused meaning and frequent inappropriate use. Others, including ourselves, consider it a useful term when applied with precision in particular contexts.

Beauchamp TL, Childress JF. *Principles of Biomedical Ethics*. 5th ed. New York: Oxford University Press; 2001:133–135, 191–194.

Zucker MB, Zucker HD, eds. *Medical Futility and the Evaluation of Life-Sustaining Interventions*. New York: Cambridge University Press; 1997.

Special Section: Medical Futility: Demands, Duties, Dilemmas. *Camb Q Healthcare Ethics* 1993;2(2):205–217.

Special Section on Futility. *J Clin Ethics* 1994;5(2):91–149.

Special Section on Futility. *J Clin Ethics* 1995;6(2):98–192.

A central ethical issue regarding probabilistic futility is whether futility should serve as a substantive norm to allow physicians to override the preferences of patients and their families or whether it should serve as a procedural norm that encourages frank discussions among physicians, patients, and their families about the appropriateness of forgoing life-sustaining treatment. In our opinion, physiologic futility constitutes a substantive norm, while probabilistic futility is a procedural norm.

Three main questions are debated about probabilistic futility: First, what level of statistical or experiential evidence is required to support a judgment of futility? Second, who decides if an intervention is futile, physicians or patients? Third, what process should be used to resolve disagreements between patients (or their surrogates) and the medical team about whether a particular treatment is futile?

(a) Statistical probability. The quantitative aspect of clinical futility requires a probabilistic judgment that an intervention is highly unlikely to produce the desired result. This judgment comes from general clinical experience and, occasionally, from clinical studies that demonstrate low rates of success for particular interventions, such as cardiopulmonary resuscitation for certain types of patients, or continued ventilatory support for patients with adult or neonatal respiratory disease syndrome. Available data about many interventions are limited, because the data provide prognostication for groups rather than for the individual. Further, a lack of agreement exists about what low level of probability would justify calling a treatment futile, and wide variation is present among experienced clinicians about what they would consider the appropriate determination of futility. One group has suggested that if soundly designed clinical studies reveal less than a 1% chance of success, intervention should be considered futile.

Schneiderman LJ, Jecker NS, Jonsen AR. Medical futility: Its meaning, and ethical implications. *Ann Intern Med* 1990;112:949–954.

EXAMPLE. A study of 865 patients who required mechanical ventilation after bone marrow transplantation showed no survivors among the 383 patients who had lung injury or hepatic or renal failure and who required more than 4 hours of ventilator support. This study suggests that it would be probabilistically futile to intubate patients with these conditions or to continue ventilation after 4 hours.

Rubenfeld GD, Crawford SW. Withdrawing life support for medically ventilated recipients of bone marrow transplantation: A case for evidence-based qualitative guidelines. *Ann Intern Med* 1996;125:625–633.

(b) Who decides? It is relatively rare that carefully designed clinical studies such as the previous reference exist for determination of futility. Inevitable debate will ensue about the level of probability that should represent futility. Who has the authority to establish the goals of the intervention and to decide the level of probability for attaining such goals? Some ethicists argue that physicians have the right to refuse care that they believe will not result in benefit; other ethicists maintain that futility must be defined in light of the subjective views, values, and goals of patients and their surrogates. This ethical debate remains unresolved, and the locus of authority for deciding futility may vary from case to case, depending on the circumstances.

Case I. A 75-year-old woman is brought to the emergency room by paramedics after suffering massive head trauma, with extrusion of brain tissue, as a result of a vehicular accident. She had been intubated by the paramedics. After careful evaluation, the emergency room physicians judged that her injuries were so severe that no intervention could retard her imminent death. When her grieving family gather in the emergency room, they demand that the woman be admitted to the ICU and be prepared for operation by a neurosurgeon. The physicians state that further treatment is futile.

Case II. Helga Wanglie was an elderly Minnesota woman who suffered irreversible brain damage from strokes and slipped into a permanent vegetative state. She required mechanical ventilation. Physicians and family agreed that she had no hope of regaining the ability to interact with others. Mrs. Wanglie's husband refused to authorize discontinuing the ventilator, saying that his goal (and, he asserted, hers) was that her life should not be shortened, regardless of her prospects for neurologic recovery. Physicians requested court intervention to authorize withdrawal of ventilatory support.

COMMENT. In Case I, the physicians use futility to designate physiologic futility, or the impossibility of continued life. They are ethically justified in refusing to pursue treatment. In Case II, continued ventilatory support and other interventions can extend Mrs. Wanglie's life. These interventions, employed for this purpose, cannot be judged physiologically futile. However, physicians judge that there is a vanishingly low probability of restoring Mrs. Wanglie's health and a low probability also that her life will be extended very long, even with support ("probabilistic futility"). They also judge that Mrs. Wanglie's life, if extended, will be of very low quality ("qualitative futility"). Physicians may recommend termination of the intervention on the grounds of probabilistic futility, but they lack the ethical authority to define the benefit as such. The benefit of continued life, even without consciousness, is a matter for the patient and her surrogate to decide (as the Minnesota court determined). Some contextual features, such as scarcity of resources, might be relevant to this case (see Chapter 4). As a matter of probabilistic and qualitative futility, which are both procedural norms, a process to resolve the disagreement among family and staff should be initiated.

(c) What process should be used to resolve disputes about futility? Institutions should design a policy for conflict resolution. These policies should prohibit unilateral decision making by physicians in cases of probabilistic and qualitative futility, stress the need for valid empirical evidence, provide for consultation with outside experts and with ethics committees, and, above all, create an atmosphere of open negotiation rather than confrontation. Futility arguments should be moved into court only after all other reasonable attempts to resolve the disagreement fail.

COMMENT. Despite continued debates about the concept of futility, it is useful in medical ethics because it highlights the necessity to make decisions about treatments that are of questionable benefit. It introduces a note of realism into excessive medical optimism by inviting physicians and families to focus on what realistically can be done for the patient under the circumstances and which patient goals, if any, can be realized. It provides the opportunity to open an honest discussion with patients and their families about appropriate care. It calls for a careful investigation of the literature about the efficacy of proposed treatments in particular situations. Physicians should never use futility, except in the sense of physiologic futility, to justify unilateral decision making or to avoid a difficult conversation with patient or family. A physician's judgment that further treatment would be probabilistically futile does not justify a conclusion that treatment should cease; instead, it signals that discussions of the situation with patient and family are mandatory. Futility should never be invoked when the real problem is a frustration with a difficult case or a reflection of the physician's negative evaluation of the patient's future quality of life (see Chapter 3). Also, a futility claim by itself does not justify rules or guidelines devised by third-party payers to avoid paying for care (see Chapter 4). Finally, even when the facts of the case support a judgment of physiologic or probabilistic futility, we suggest that it may be advisable to avoid the actual word "futility" in discussions with patients or their families. Many persons may interpret this word as an announcement that the physician is "giving up" on the patient. We suggest that the futility situation be discussed in terms of the principle of proportionality, that is, the imbalance of expected benefits over burdens imposed by continued interventions (see Section 3.2.4).

1.1.4 Patients with Progressive, Lethal Disease

Certain diseases follow a course of gradual and sometimes occult destruction of the body's physiologic processes. Patients who suffer such diseases may experience their effects continually or intermittently and with varying severity. Eventually, the disease itself or some associated disorder will cause their death. Mrs. Care illustrates the features of this condition. Multiple sclerosis cannot be cured; progressive neurologic complications that include spasticity, loss of mobility, neurogenic bladder, respiratory insufficiency, and occasionally dementia are also incurable. Still, some interventions, such as treatment of infection, can relieve symptoms, maintain some level of function, and prolong life.

Case. For the first decade after her diagnosis with MS, Mrs. Care maintained high spirits. Although she did not like to discuss her disease or its prognosis, she seemed to understand the progressive and lethal nature of her condition. However, in the last few years, she has begun to speak frequently of "getting this over," and has become deeply depressed. She has accepted several trials of antidepressant medications, but these did not improve her mental condition. As serious urinary tract and respiratory infections became more frequent, she grudgingly submitted to treatment.

COMMENT. Patients in this condition are not terminal, even though the disease from which they suffer is incurable. However, they may from time to time experience acute, critical episodes, which, if not treated, would lead to their death. When successfully treated, patients will be restored to their "baseline condition." In a sense, they are, at each episode, "potentially terminal." It may occur to such patients and to their physicians that these episodes offer an opportunity to end their progressive decline. Recall the old medical maxim, "Pneumonia is the old person's friend." In such a situation, the issues require a careful review of medical indications because the patient's prognosis, with or without treatment, must be clearly understood. However, the more important questions concern patient preferences and quality of life. Thus, the ethical dimensions of such cases will be discussed in Chapters 2 and 3.

1.1 P Decisions to Forgo Futile Interventions for Children

With infants and children, as with adults, recommendations must sometimes be made about the appropriate forms of care when death appears imminent. Although it is often psychologically and emotionally more difficult to accept the death of an infant or child, pediatricians must sometimes recommend that certain interventions are not medically indicated because they are futile, providing no or only minimal benefits, or because they impose burdens disproportionate to their benefits. All of the cautions about the concept of futility mentioned previously should be observed. The statement earlier (Section 1.1.3) about the use of the word "futility" in discussions with patients and family is even more appropriate when discussing with parents the futility of interventions for their child. Framing the discussion in the principle of proportionality is advisable (see Section 3.2.4).

Case I. A fetus is delivered by spontaneous abortion at 21 weeks of gestation, weighing 350 g, and is asphyxiated at birth.

Case II. Jason, a 4-year-old boy, absent from home for about 2 hours, is found at the bottom of a next-door swimming pool. When drawn from the water, he is limp, with grayish pallor, and cold. His father initiates mouth-to-mouth resuscitation with no response. The emergency service arrives 8 minutes later. During the ambulance trip to the emergency room, cardiopulmonary resuscitation for 26 minutes and two doses of epinephrine fail to stimulate any physiologic response. Rectal temperature is 35°C.

Case III. Kerry was born at 23 weeks of gestation weighing 590 g. In the delivery room, she required intubation and ventilation; Apgar scores were 2 at 1 minute and 5 at 5 minutes. Kerry had severe hyaline membrane disease and was started on surfactant replacement. Initially in 80% oxygen with high-pressure ventilator settings, Kerry was weaned down to 30% oxygen. Kerry's anterior fontanel was noted to be tense, and a head ultrasound revealed a bilateral grade IV intracerebral hemorrhage with associated periventricular leukomalacia. On the fifth day of life,

Kerry had surgery for removal of a necrotic small bowel from the pylorus to the large colon. The infant then developed candidal sepsis.

Case IV. Amy was diagnosed with acute myelogenous leukemia (AML) at the age of 8 years. She received a course of chemotherapy, resulting in a remission after 6 months. Three months later she relapsed. An allogeneic bone marrow transplantation was performed with her 17-year-old sister as a compatible donor. Again, after several months, Amy's cancer returned. Her parents requested more chemotherapy, which her oncologist advised would be very unlikely to succeed. Despite a course of experimental chemotherapy, Amy's disease progressed. After 2 difficult months, Amy, who had been a cheerful patient, became very discouraged. Her parents and her sister urged her to continue the experimental regimen. Amy, now aged 10 years, asks why she "has to keep doing this?"

COMMENT. In all the above cases, it is reasonable to judge that interventions to sustain organic functions will be incapable of restoring these functions to independent activity. In Case I, no infant of that birth weight and gestational age is known to have survived under current medical regimens. Although this may constitute probabilistic futility, it more likely reflects the physiologic incapacity of immature lungs to perform their essential work and thus would constitute physiologic futility. In Case II, resuscitative efforts can be discontinued on grounds of probabilistic futility. Current data suggest that failure to get a physiologic response after more than 20 minutes of resuscitative efforts and two doses of epinephrine justifies termination of interventions. In the unlikely event that resuscitation succeeds, Jason has probably sustained brain damage that would severely compromise the quality of his future life. In Case III, Kerry's lung disease has improved somewhat with surfactant and may continue to improve, even to the point of discontinuing respiratory support. Neurologic function and alimentary tract are badly damaged; surgical loss of such extensive bowel seriously compromises survival. The probability of surviving candidal infection is remote. Thus, given this complex of problems, a general assessment of probabilistic futility is reasonable. In Case IV, further treatment has only the most remote probability of attaining remission and none of cure, thereby justifying the physician's recommendation not to proceed with further chemotherapy. In addition, Amy's emotional response to the prospect of further treatment should be respected, as discussed in Chapter 2.

RECOMMENDATION. In all these cases, reasonable judgments of physiologic or probabilistic futility can be made. Such judgments are a sound justification for a decision to discontinue medical interventions or not to

intervene. In such cases, physicians should recommend that nonbenefi-
cial treatments be withheld or withdrawn. This recommendation must
be expressed with great sensitivity, because parents often cannot accept
the fact of their child's inevitable death. Should parents reject this recommendation, the comments at Section 2.7 P are relevant.

Case V. Patrick was born at 35 weeks of gestation after his mother went
into premature labor precipitated by polyhydramnios. A prenatal ultrasound, done at 22 weeks of gestation, demonstrated a left-sided diaphragmatic hernia. Vigorous at birth, Patrick was immediately intubated and ventilated because of the rapid onset of cyanosis and
respiratory distress. In spite of high pressures on the ventilator and
100% oxygen, Patrick's arterial oxygen never went above 60 mm Hg nor
did his carbon dioxide go below 50 mm Hg. Inhaled nitric oxide and
high-frequency ventilation failed to improve oxygenation and ventilation. A chest radiograph showed that Patrick had a large hernia with
stomach, intestine, and liver located in his left thorax. His right lung also
appeared hypoplastic. The neonatologists considered extracorporeal
membrane oxygenation (ECMO).

COMMENT. ECMO is used as therapy for severe pulmonary hypertension.
It is a procedure whereby blood is diverted out of the body and the infant's oxygenation and ventilation are supported while vessels of the
lungs progressively relax. ECMO has improved the survival of infants
with pulmonary hypertension. However, with diaphragmatic hernia,
both lungs are underdeveloped and thus may not support normal oxygenation and ventilation even with ECMO. Although there are currently
no certain predictors that discriminate between those who will benefit
from ECMO and those who will not, prematurity, gestational age at diagnosis, and extent of lung hypoplasia seem significant. In Patrick's case,
a judgment of probabilistic futility is reasonable. In cases of this sort, it
is emotionally difficult for physicians and family to acknowledge futility,
because technology seems to encourage even futile efforts in the face of
certain death.

Case VI. At 24 weeks of gestation, a fetus was diagnosed by ultrasound
as having severe diaphragmatic hernia. Most of the abdominal viscera
were herniated into the left chest, and there was almost no visible lung.

COMMENT. Diaphragmatic hernia of this severity is thought to be incompatible with postnatal life. There are four options for the management of
this fetus: (1) terminate the pregnancy; (2) no supportive care after birth,
allowing early death; (3) aggressive postnatal care, including respiratory
support, ECMO, and surgical correction; and (4) immediate fetal surgi-

cal repair. Postnatal care will be in all likelihood futile, because the child will have almost no lung to support respiratory function. Fetal surgical repair is theoretically the most efficacious approach, but is experimental and should be chosen only in light of the criteria for clinical research, as discussed in Chapter 4.

1.2 ORDERS NOT TO ATTEMPT RESUSCITATION

One form of medical intervention, cardiopulmonary resuscitation (CPR), deserves careful attention under the topic of indications for medical intervention. Cardiopulmonary resuscitation consists of a set of techniques designed to restore circulation and respiration in the event of acute cardiac or cardiopulmonary arrest. CPR, in its simplest form of mouth-to-mouth insufflation and chest compression, is taught to lay persons for use in emergency situations. In hospitals, advanced CPR is usually done by a trained team who respond to an urgent call. Advanced CPR techniques include closed-chest compression, intubation with assisted ventilation, electroconversion of arrhythmias, defibrillation, and cardiotonic and vasopressive drugs.

The Joint Commission of Health Care Organizations requires that hospitals have a formal policy regarding CPR. Usually, those policies will require that CPR is a standing order; that is, it is to be performed without a specific order on any patient who suffers a cardiac or respiratory arrest. Only when a specific order is issued that CPR is not to be done may it be omitted. This order is called Do Not Attempt Resuscitation (DNAR) and is frequently designated as a "No Code Order." The omission of CPR after cardiopulmonary arrest will result in the death of the patient. A DNAR order may be considered a form of advance planning that permits patients to die peacefully without the rigors of resuscitative attempts.

The decision to write a DNAR order is a complex one. Three crucial considerations must be assessed. The first is the judgment that CPR would be futile, that is, that the resuscitation would be very unlikely to succeed or, if it did, the patient would not survive to be discharged from the hospital. The second important aspect of DNAR concerns the preferences of the patient, if known, and the third pertains to the expected quality of life of the patient for whom resuscitation succeeds. The first aspect, the medical futility of the intervention will be treated here; patient preferences and quality of life will be discussed in Chapters 2 and 3. All three aspects must be assessed in any decision to write a DNAR order.

1.2.1 Medical Indications and Contraindications for CPR

All persons who suffer unexpected cardiopulmonary arrest for a known or unknown cause and who are not known to be terminally and irreversibly ill should be resuscitated. This is made clear in the standards for CPR:

> The purpose of cardiopulmonary resuscitation is the prevention of sudden, unexpected death. Cardiopulmonary resuscitation is not indicated in certain situations, such as in cases of terminal, irreversible illness where death is not unexpected.
>
> Standards and guidelines for cardiopulmonary resuscitation (CPR) and emergency cardiac care (ECC). *JAMA* 1980;244:453–509.

COMMENT. (a) Cardiopulmonary resuscitation is inappropriate medical practice in the case of cardiopulmonary arrest that occurs as the anticipated end of a terminal illness or after maximal efforts to save the patient have failed. For such patients, a DNAR order should be written.

(b) DNAR orders are usually first considered when the patient is in a terminal condition and death appears to be imminent. A multicenter study of DNAR orders written in ICUs showed that fewer than 2% of patients who had DNAR orders survived to be discharged from the hospital. Increasingly, however, nonterminally ill patients, many of whom are in the earlier phases of diseases, such as metastatic cancer and AIDS, but who are not moribund or acutely terminally ill, discuss DNAR orders with their physicians as a component of advanced care planning. Many of these patients are prepared to forego resuscitation attempts because they are concerned that even if they are "successfully" resuscitated, they may experience anoxic brain damage or some other functional impairment. For seriously ill patients who have DNAR orders, several published studies have shown survival to discharge to be as high as 50% to 70%.

(c) In the United States, the rate of DNAR orders varies from 3% to 30% among hospitalized patients and between 5% and 20% among patients admitted to ICUs. Sixty-six percent to 75% of hospital deaths and 40% of deaths in ICUs are preceded by a DNAR order. Even after adjusting for severity of illness, disparities exist in the use of DNAR orders relative to age, race, gender, and geography. Older patients, white patients, and men are more likely to have DNAR orders. Some geographic areas have a DNAR rate 8 to 10 times higher than others.

(d) The rationale for DNAR orders varies greatly, but in general, these orders are written for three reasons: patient preferences, poor prognosis and age greater than 75 years (regardless of prognosis).

SUPPORT Principal Investigators. A controlled trial to improve care for seriously ill hospitalized patients. *JAMA* 1995;274:1591–1598.

(e) Studies also indicate that even for terminally ill patients, DNAR orders are underused (as measured by the number of patients who had indicated a preference for such orders in relation to those for whom orders were actually written) because of a lack of communication and discussion among physicians, patients, and their families. In our view, it is the responsibility of physicians to initiate DNAR discussions in the following situations: (1) DNAR discussions should be held with patients capable of making decisions (or with the surrogates of patients who are incapable of making decisions) if they are terminally ill or have an incurable disease with an estimated 50% survival of less than 3 years; (2) DNAR discussions should be held with all patients who suffer acute, life-threatening conditions; and (3) DNAR discussions should be held with patients who request such a discussion.

(f) Recent studies have shown that CPR is not effective in restoring cardiac function for certain classes of patients or has only a low probability of being successful. Even when CPR succeeded at the time of the arrest, fewer than 15% of these patients survived to discharge. Survival was more likely in the following situations: (1) for patients with respiratory rather than cardiac arrest; (2) for witnessed cardiac arrests, initial ventricular tachycardia, or fibrillation; (3) for patients with no or few comorbid conditions; and (4) for patients who experienced a short duration of CPR. Survival is much less likely in patients with preexisting hypotension, renal failure, sepsis, pneumonia, acute stroke, metastatic cancer, or a homebound lifestyle. For the small percentage of patients who survive to discharge, several studies have shown good long-term prognosis, with survival rates of 33% to 54%. It is essential that patients, their families, and physicians have this kind of information on the benefits and risks of CPR so that they can make informed decisions about using CPR or choosing DNAR status.

(g) Competent patients sometimes request that DNAR orders be issued, and physicians should comply with such a request to honor the patient's preferences. At least one state court has determined that resuscitation against a patient-requested DNAR order does not create civil liability in the noncomplying physician. The court noted, however, that the physician could be liable for any direct harm caused to the patient as a result of the attempted resuscitation, and that the physician may be subject to sanctions by licensing boards.

Anderson v St. Francis-St. George (Ohio, 1996).

Other states may impose liability in such a situation, and, regardless of the state of the law, the physician has an ethical duty to honor the patient's preference to not be resuscitated.

1.2.2 Unilateral DNAR Orders

Ordinarily, the consent of the patient or the patient's surrogate to forgo CPR is required. However, medical ethicists are currently debating whether it is ever ethically acceptable for a physician to make a unilateral decision, that is, a decision not to resuscitate without consulting the patient or the patient's surrogate, or even in the face of objections from the patient or surrogate. Those in favor of unilateral decisions argue that a medical judgment that CPR would be futile means that it is not indicated; that is, it would not attain the goals of medicine and thus need not be offered as an option to the patient. Those who reject this position argue that it violates the standard of informed consent. The patient should always have the right to refuse or choose CPR, because a decision about the goals of treatment and the acceptable probability of attaining those goals is a judgment that the patient should make. Even the remote chance of successful resuscitation may be of value to the patient. Further, these ethicists note that a lack of agreement exists on what level of survival probability constitutes futility and that physicians are inconsistent in their application of the futility concept. Finally, unilateral decisions are open to bias against racial minorities and other patients who might be subjected to discrimination.

COMMENT. If the physician has concluded that CPR would be physiologically futile, the order may be given unilaterally. For example, the patient is exsanguinated on arrival in the Emergency Department and has been pulseless with a flat ECG for 20 minutes. When the patient is terminal but not moribund, we recommend, that consent be sought from available surrogates. If they refuse, the policy should include the following four mandatory provisions: (1) The physician must obtain a second opinion; (2) the hospital ethics committee must be consulted; (3) an atmosphere for negotiation between parties must be created; and (4) the patient's right to be transferred to another provider must be preserved.

EXAMPLES. (a) Mr. Cure, the young man with severe headache and stiff neck, is admitted to the hospital with a diagnosis of meningitis. He refuses antibiotic therapy. Within a few minutes, he suffers a cardiac arrest. The intern, aware of the patient's refusal of necessary therapy, wonders whether resuscitation should be initiated.

(b) Mrs. Care, the patient with multiple sclerosis, has been admitted to the hospital in coma for treatment of pneumonia and respiratory failure. In the past, she has emphasized to her family and physicians that she did not wish to be placed on permanent mechanical ventilation. Neurologic consultation concludes that her respiratory insufficiency is secondary to the advancing muscular and neurologic deterioration of MS and that respiratory failure was accelerated by her acute pneumonia. Should a DNAR be written?

(c) L.M., a 68-year-old man without family, has been diagnosed with critical aortic stenosis (0.3-mm orifice) and scheduled for immediate valvuloplasty. On emerging from his doctor's office, he suffers a cardiac arrest. No discussion of CPR has taken place. Should he be resuscitated?

RECOMMENDATIONS. Mr. Cure, even though he has refused antibiotic therapy for a life-threatening condition, should certainly be resuscitated. The reason for his refusal has not been adequately elucidated, and the refusal of a particular therapy should not be taken as equivalent to refusal of all therapy. Failure to resuscitate would constitute serious medical negligence and ethical fault. In the case of Mrs. Care, recommendations should be made to the family that even if CPR succeeds, the patient would survive only a short time without permanent ventilatory support. If the patient's prior wishes not to be intubated are known to the medical team, and if the family concurs, a DNAR order should be entered. If the family disagrees, CPR should be provided in the event of a cardiac arrest. Mr. L.M. may exemplify "physiologic futility." His aortic stenosis is very severe. Patients in this situation have a fixed cardiac output that cannot be improved by the usual procedures of CPR. Although immediate catheterization might be temporarily effective, his arrest has taken place about 30 minutes from the nearest catheterization facility. His physician might also immediately administer an alpha-agonist, but if there is no response, he might reasonably refrain from further resuscitative attempts on grounds of physiologic futility.

1.2.3 Documentation of DNAR Orders

Attending physicians should clearly write and sign the DNAR in the orders section of the patient's chart. The progress notes should include the medical facts and opinion underlying the order and a summary of the discussion with the patient, consultants, staff, and family. The status of the order should be reviewed at regular intervals in view of the condition of the patient and should be changed when the condition of the patient warrants it. Everyone involved with the care of the patient should be informed of the DNAR order and its rationale. Because studies have shown that DNAR means different things to different practitioners, the physician writing the order must be careful to document the specific terms of the order. Decisions to withhold or withdraw interventions other than DNAR should be noted by the writing of specific orders rather than relying on the DNAR order to cover a wide range of decisions. The writing of a DNAR order should have no direct bearing on any treatment other than CPR. Physicians should recall that many patients for whom DNAR orders are written survive to be discharged from the hospital. If the patient is readmitted, a DNAR order that is in the patient's chart from a previous admission should be reviewed with the patient and surrogate and in light of medical indications.

1.2.4 DNAR Portability

Patients for whom DNAR orders have been written in the hospital may be discharged with the expectation that they will die soon. Often, patients want to die in their own homes rather than in the hospital. It sometimes happens that these patients suffer a crisis at home and family members summon emergency services. Traditionally, emergency medical service providers, because of the time constraints inherent in emergency services, were not held responsible for determining whether a patient has executed an advanced directive. They attempt to resuscitate all patients regardless of the patients' preferences. In recent years, a method of protecting an individual's preference not to be resuscitated has been devised. This is called a "portable" DNAR. These are orders issued by the patient's discharging physician, stated in a standard form, and indicated on bracelets, necklaces, or wallet cards. When the patient has this order, providers are authorized to refrain from CPR, although all other necessary treatments can still be provided. Forty-four states now have laws mandating that EMS providers comply with out-of-hospital DNARs. Once the emergency care provider has verified that the order appears valid and that the patient is the person who has executed it, the provider cannot commence CPR except in certain circumstances, such as when the patient renounces the document.

1.2.5 "Partial Codes" and "Slow Codes"

The infamous "slow code" (sometimes called "show," "light blue," or "Hollywood code") describes a subterfuge in which doctors and nurses respond slowly to a cardiac arrest and perform CPR without energy or enthusiasm, simply to show the family that something is being done. This is done usually in two circumstances: (1) when the medical team feels that resuscitation would be futile, but no discussion has taken place with the patient or the family, or (2) when the family has chosen resuscitation, and the team feels it would be useless. Clinical experience suggests that patients rarely, if ever, are successfully resuscitated by a slow code. A slow code is dishonest, crass dissimulation, and unethical.

Occasionally, one hears the expression "partial code." This refers to the practice of separating the various interventions that constitute resuscitation and using them selectively; thus, chest compression, assisted breathing by AMBU bag, and cardiotonic drugs may be ordered, but intubation may be omitted. CPR may be defined as an integrated set of procedures, all of which should be applied to reverse all the effects of cardiac arrest. Still, with sufficient and clear rationale, physicians and patients may develop a plan for resuscitation that omits one or another intervention. For example, a terminal patient may tell the doctor that if his heart stops, he would want the doctor to start it again but would not want to be intubated.

1.2.6 DNAR Orders in the Operating Room

Patients may suffer a cardiac arrest in the course of, or as the result of, a medical intervention. In such cases, even when there is no medical error, physicians can be seen as the agents of this adverse event. Surgical procedures may be the occasion of an iatrogenic cardiac arrest. Occasionally, patients for whom a DNAR order has been written, such as patients with terminal cancer, may require a palliative surgical procedure, such as emergency correction of a bowel obstruction to relieve pain or the elective insertion of a gastrostomy tube or a central venous catheter. Physicians have questioned whether the DNAR order should be suspended automatically during anesthesia or surgery, so that the patients would be resuscitated if they experienced a perioperative cardiac arrest. The arguments favoring this policy are (1) anesthesia and surgery place patients at risk for cardiac and hemodynamic instability; (2) most arrests in the operating room are reversible, because skilled personnel and equipment are at hand; (3) in consenting to surgery, the patient gives implied consent for resuscitation; and (4) surgeons and anesthesiologists should not be prevented from treating potentially reversible situations, especially because they do not wish deaths of terminally ill patients to be considered surgical deaths when standard resuscitative techniques have been prohibited. In one study, the majority of anesthesiologists assumed that DNAR was implicitly suspended during surgery, and only half of anesthesiologists discussed this assumption with the patient or surrogate.

Those opposed to automatic suspension of DNAR orders note that such a policy ignores patients' rights and violates the standards of informed consent. They recommend instead a policy of "required reconsideration." The patient who consents to elective surgery faces a different risk versus benefit situation, and this merits a reevaluation of the DNAR order. A specific discussion about DNAR should occur between the attending physicians and surgeons and the patient or surrogates and should either affirm or suspend the order in anticipation of surgery. The major professional associations of surgeons, anesthesiologists, and nurses have endorsed this policy, and we recommend it as the most prudent course. We also advise that if a competent patient, after reconsideration, wishes a preexisting DNAR order to stand, resuscitation should not be attempted in the event of an intrasurgical arrest.

Statement of the American College of Surgeons. Advanced Directive by Patients: Do Not Resuscitate in the Operating Room. *Bull Am Coll Surg* 1994;79(9):29.

Another approach to this problem is to develop DNAR orders that list the goals of the patient and that permit the surgeon and anesthesiologist to use their clinical judgment to try to achieve the patient's goals. Thus, if the patient fears anoxic brain damage and experiences ventricular tachycardia that is promptly corrected by cardioversion, the patient's goals will be met. Alternatively, if the patient experiences 15 or more minutes of cardiac arrest, secondary to an intraoperative MI, the surgeon and anesthesiologist may stop CPR to respect the patient's wish not to survive with neurologic damage.

1.2 P Orders Not to Resuscitate Infants and Children

In general, the conditions for an order not to initiate cardiopulmonary resuscitation are the same for a child as for an adult, with the exception of the patient's consent. However, resuscitation of the asphyxiated newborn raises special questions.

Case I. A baby is delivered by spontaneous abortion at 23 weeks of gestation, weighing 410 g, and is asphyxiated at birth.

Case II. An infant, born at 33 weeks of gestation, appears to be microcephalic, with low-set, posteriorly rotated ears. A single umbilical artery is noted, in addition to an oddly shaped chest. The birth had been precipitous, the mother having received meperidine IM 1 hour preceding. Apgar score is 1 at 1 minute; heart rate is 80 beats/min.

COMMENT AND RECOMMENDATION. Decisions made in the delivery room are not true examples of DNAR orders, because no order is written before the need for resuscitation. In these cases, the necessity for resuscitation may be assessed at the time of delivery. However, given contemporary prenatal evaluation, the need may be assessed before delivery, thereby prompting discussion of whether resuscitation should be attempted at delivery. In Case I, it is ethically correct to determine before birth or at birth not to resuscitate. Experience indicates that even if resuscitated, this very small premature infant will not survive. In Case II, resuscitation should be attempted, because the nature of the child's congenital problems is not clear, and the depressed state of the infant is possibly due to the presence of narcotics. Resuscitation and evaluation do not rule out a later decision to withdraw treatment, on the basis of either medical indications or quality-of-life considerations, as discussed in Chapter 3.

1.3 CARE OF THE DYING PATIENT

The decision to terminate specific forms of treatment or not to resuscitate does not imply the termination of care for the patient. It is frequently noted that after a DNAR order is written, attention to the patient's needs diminishes. This is unethical for two reasons. First, in some series more than 50% of patients for whom DNAR orders have been written survive to be discharged. These patients require continued appropriate care. Second, it is a failure to recognize that, when the goals of curing are exhausted, the goals of caring must be reinforced. Attention to relief of pain and discomfort and enhancement of the patient's ability to interact with family and friends become predominant goals. The medical proverb is pertinent: Cure sometimes, relieve occasionally, comfort always. Particular issues in the care of the dying patient, such as pain control, are discussed in Chapter 3.

1.4 LEGAL IMPLICATIONS OF FORGOING TREATMENT

It might be claimed that forgoing a medical intervention constitutes an act of negligence, and the death of a patient resulting from such negligence would constitute homicide. It is a general principle of the law of medical negligence that the testimony of expert witnesses that a particular medical intervention is not indicated stands as a defense against a charge of negligence. Thus, if expert witnesses affirm that some intervention would be judged futile, presumably physicians are safe to recommend that it be omitted. Although many judicial decisions have supported the decision to discontinue life support or to order DNAR, most of these rely on legal interpretations of patients' preferences and on the patients' quality of life rather than on claims of medical futility alone. We list the most important of these cases in Chapter 3. Two recent cases pertain more directly to futility. In the Wanglie case, discussed previously at Section 1.1.3, Case II, the court supported a surrogate's demand to continue ventilator support for an 87-year-old woman in a persistent vegetative state, although the attending physicians considered it medically inappropriate (In re Wanglie, Minn., 1991). In the Gilgunn case, a jury trial held the hospital harmless against claims of the family for discontinuing care judged futile by attending physicians whose judgment was endorsed by the hospital's ethics committee.

Gilgunn v Massachusetts General Hospital (Mass. 1995).

Neither case provides clear guidance for practitioners. We recommend that hospitals formulate policy defining appropriate care and stating the methods whereby decisions in difficult cases should be made and reviewed. Physicians and hospitals are most justifiably criticized and most likely to get into difficulty when they make unilateral decisions, especially if they have failed to communicate and negotiate with surrogates, consult with colleagues, follow administrative procedures and policies, or seek legal consultation.

1.4 P Legal Implications of Forgoing Life Support for Children

In 1985, the U.S. Congress passed amendments to The Child Abuse Prevention and Treatment and Adoption Reform Act, which pertain to clinical decisions about newborns. The regulations based on this legislation are known as the "Baby Doe Rules." These rules are discussed at Section 4.6 P. However, here we note only that the rules do not require life-sustaining treatment, "when the provision of such treatment would merely prolong dying, not be effective in ameliorating or correcting all of the infant's life threatening conditions, or otherwise be futile in terms of the survival of the infant."

45 Code of Federal Regulations 1340, April 15, 1985.

One controversial court decision, known as the case of Baby K., is also discussed at Section 4.6 P. That case seems to imply that even irreversibly dying infants are entitled to emergency lifesaving care if a parent demands such care. Given the circumstances of the case, the ruling cannot be generalized and clinicians should seek legal counsel about its interpretation.

1.5 DETERMINATION OF DEATH

Medical intervention ceases when the patient is declared dead. Declaring death is one of the legal duties of physicians. Traditionally, the moment of death was considered to be the time when a person ceased, and did not resume, communication, movement, and breathing. The body soon becomes cold and rigid, and putrefaction sets in. It became customary for physicians to determine death by noting the absence of respiration and pulse and the fixation of pupils. Thus, the common definition of death, accepted in medicine and in the law, was "irreversible cessation of circulation and respiration." This is known as the "cardiorespiratory criterion" of death.

This criterion presupposes loss of the integrating function of the brainstem. When this function ceases, spontaneous breathing stops, followed by a disintegration of all vital organ systems. The unoxygenated brain rapidly loses all cognitive and other regulatory functions; the unoxygenated heart ceases to beat. In the 1960s, it became possible to maintain respiratory functions by the use of a mechanical ventilator, which can support oxygen perfusion even in the absence of brainstem function.

The concept of "brain criteria" for death that would complement or replace "cardiorespiratory criteria" emerged in the 1960s. The advent of organ transplantation stimulated interest in this concept, because its application would make possible the preservation of organs after death. In 1968, the document indicated below was published.

Report of the Ad Hoc Committee of the Harvard Medical School to Examine the Definition of Brain Death, "A Definition of Irreversible Coma." *N Eng J Med* 1968;205:337.

This report described certain clinical characteristics of a person with a nonfunctioning brain: unreceptivity and unresponsivity to external stimuli, no movements or breathing, no reflexes, and no discernible electrical activity in the cerebral cortex as shown by electroencephalogram (EEG).

The use of "brain criteria" for determination of clinical death was gradually accepted by legal jurisdictions. However, much confusion existed about their proper application. In particular, confusion existed between "total brain death" and "irreversible coma" (now called "persistent vegetative state," (see Section 3.2.2). This confusion was the source of ethical and legal problems. Thus, in 1981, the President's Commission for the Study of Ethical Problems in Medicine proposed a model legal statute, The Uniform Definition of Death (UDDA). As of 1999, every state and the District of Columbia now accepts the brain death criteria either by statute or judicial decision.

An individual who has sustained either (1) irreversible cessation of circulatory and respiratory function, or (2) irreversible cessation of all functions of the entire brain, including the brain stem, is dead. A determination of death must be made in accordance with accepted medical standards.

President's Commission on Ethical Problems in Medicine and Biomedical and Behavioral Research. *Defining Death: A Report on the Medical, Legal, and Ethical Issues in Definition of Death.* Washington, DC: Government Printing Office; 1981.

The accepted medical standards for clinical diagnosis of death by brain criteria are as follows: after ruling out confounding conditions such as drug intoxication and severe hypothermia, it should be demonstrated that there are no voluntary or involuntary movements except spinal reflexes and no brainstem reflexes (eg, apnea in the presence of elevated arterial CO_2 when mechanical ventilation is temporarily halted, fixed and dilated pupils, fixed at midposition, no reaction to aural irrigation, no gag reflex). Brain blood-flow studies are confirmatory. Electroencephalography, which diagnoses only absence of cortical function, is not sufficient to establish total brain death and is frequently omitted in the presence of the above clinical signs.

No medical goals are attainable for a person who is dead by either cardiorespiratory criteria or brain criteria. All interventions should be terminated. The physician has the authority to declare the patient dead; there is no legal or ethical requirement to seek permission from the family to declare a patient dead or to discontinue medical interventions. The family should be sensitively informed that their relative has died. Contextual features of a particular case might suggest a continuation of supportive technology, for example, sensitivity to needs of family and friends of the patient, salvage of a viable fetus from a brain-dead pregnant woman, or retrieval of organs for transplant (see Chapter 4).

It is particularly important that physicians distinguish the ethical and legal implications of death by brain criteria from the implications of the persistent vegetative state. Lay persons (and some physicians and nurses) use the term "brain death" when they are referring to persistent vegetative state. This is wrong. The ethical and legal implications of persistent vegetative state are discussed at Section 3.2.2.

Certain philosophical problems about the adequacy of the definition of death by brain criteria remain open to debate. These disputes need not concern those responsible for clinical decisions in this matter. At the present time, physicians in every legal jurisdiction can rely on the legal, clinical, and ethical determinations mentioned earlier. Religious denominations have generally accepted this definition of death. The notable exception is Orthodox Judaism, where many authorities insist on use of the cardiorespiratory criteria for theological reasons.

1.5 P Determination of Death for Children

The clinical method of determining death by brain criteria may be used for infants and children, but special caution is advised, because it is assumed, although not proven, that the child's brain is more resistant to insults leading to death. Physicians responsible for making this determination in children should be familiar with the special clinical issues. In addition to the general criteria (eg, coma, apnea, absence of brainstem function demonstrated by nonreactive pupils, absence of eye movement, flaccid tone, no spontaneous movement other than spinal cord reflexes, and a ruling-out of hypothermia and hypotension), studies that are only confirmatory in adults are advised, that is, EEG and cerebral blood-flow studies. An observation period of at least 48 hours is recommended. Naturally, the greatest sympathy and understanding must be extended to parents whose children have died. It is particularly important to make clear that death by brain criteria is distinct from persistent vegetative condition; the term "brain death" confuses the two and should be avoided. Similarly, pediatricians should not speak of "removing life support" when ventilators are supporting breathing after a determination of death by brain criteria. The child is not living and thus the ventilator is not supporting life. Such language only reinforces the mistaken notion that the parents have "let their child die" by authorizing removal of ventilatory support.

Task Force on Brain Death in Children. Guidelines for the determination of brain death in children. *Pediatrics* 1987;80:298–299.

Chapter 2

2.0 ▪ ▪ ▪ ▪ ▪ ▪ ▪ ▪ ▪ ▪ ▪ ▪ ▪

Preferences of Patients

This chapter discusses the second topic that is essential to the analysis of an ethical problem in clinical medicine, namely, the Preferences of Patients. The first topic, medical indications, concerns the clinical judgment of the physician that leads to a recommendation to the patient or designated surrogate about an appropriate course of care. This chapter will discuss the issues associated with the expression or the absence of patient preferences in the following order: (1) ethical, legal, clinical, and psychologic significance of patient preferences; (2) informed consent; (3) decisional capacity; (4) truth in medical communication; (5) cultural and religious beliefs; (6) refusal of treatment; (7) advance directives; (8) surrogate decisions; (9) the uncooperative patient; and (10) alternative medicine.

When there are medical indications for treatment, a physician should propose a treatment plan that a competent patient may accept or refuse. An informed, competent patient's preference to accept or to refuse medically indicated treatment has clinical, ethical, legal, and psychologic importance. Patient preferences are the ethical and legal nucleus of a patient-physician relationship; in most circumstances, the relationship can neither be initiated nor sustained unless the patient desires it. Even though the patient may need the assistance of a physician, the patient, not the physician, has the primary legal and moral authority to establish the relationship.

2.0.1 Clinical Significance of Patient Preferences

Knowledge of patient preferences is essential to good clinical care, because the patient's cooperation and satisfaction reflect the degree to which medical intervention fulfills the patient's choices, values, and needs. Patients who collaborate with their physicians to reach a shared health care decision have greater trust and loyalty in the doctor-patient relationship, cooperate more fully to implement the shared decision, and express greater satisfaction with their health care. Most importantly, such patients have now been shown to have better clinical outcomes in at least the following four chronic conditions: hypertension, non-insulin-dependent diabetes mellitus, peptic ulcer disease, and rheumatoid arthritis. As medicine has become more effective, a particular problem can often be treated by several medically reasonable options, and each option is associated with different risks and benefits for the patient. For example, to avoid the risk of perioperative death, some patients with lung cancer may choose radiation therapy over surgery despite a lower 5-year survival rate. Similarly, some patients may choose prophylactic mastectomy over watchful waiting when told they have a strong genetic susceptibility to breast cancer or may choose watchful waiting over surgery for symptomatic benign prostatic hypertrophy.

Different patients may express different but entirely reasonable preferences when faced with the same medical indications. Some physicians are more likely than others to invite the expression of patient preferences and to encourage a "participatory decision-making style." Research has shown that patients with chronic diseases enjoy better health outcomes when they ask questions, express opinions, and make their preferences known, and when their physicians have a "participatory" rather than a "controlling" decision-making style. A participatory style is associated with primary care training, skill in interviewing that facilitates empathic listening and communication, and the opportunity to take time with patients.

2.0.2 Ethical Significance of Patient Preferences: Autonomy

Patient preferences are ethically significant because they manifest the value of personal autonomy that is deeply rooted in the ethics of our culture. Moral philosophers emphasize the principle of autonomy, the moral right to choose and follow one's own plan of life and action. **Respect for autonomy** is the moral attitude that disposes one to refrain from interference with the autonomous beliefs and actions of others in the pursuit of their goals. Constraint of a person's free choices is morally permissible only when one person's preferences and actions seriously infringe on the rights and welfare of another. The recognition of patient preferences respects the value of personal autonomy in medical care. In practice, however, many forces obstruct and limit the expression and appreciation of patient preferences. These forces—for example, the compromised competence of the patient, the disparity between the practitioner's knowledge and that of the patient, the psychodynamics of the patient-physician relationship, and the stress of illness—often make difficult the realization of respect for the autonomy of the patient.

Beauchamp TL, Childress JF. Respect for autonomy. In: *Principles of Biomedical Ethics*. 5th ed. New York: Oxford University Press; 2001:57–103.

2.0.3 Legal Significance of Patient Preferences: Self-Determination

Patient preferences are legally significant because the American legal system recognizes that all persons have a fundamental right to control their own body and the right to be protected from unwanted intrusions or "unconsented touchings." Two classic judicial opinions state this principle frankly and succinctly:

> Every human being of adult years and of sound mind has a right to determine what shall be done with his body.
>
> *Schloendorff v Society of New York Hospital*, (N.Y. 1914).

> Anglo-American law starts with the premise of thoroughgoing self-determination. It follows that each man is considered to be master of his own body, and he may, if he be of sound mind, prohibit the performance of life-saving surgery or other medical treatment.
>
> *Natanson v Kline*, (Kan. 1960).

The legal requirement of explicit consent before specific treatment protects the legal right of patients to control what is done to their own bodies. The documentation of the patient's consent also serves as a defense for the physician against a claim that the patient was coerced. Finally, apart from clinical skill and carefulness, a respect for patient preferences, good communication, and a participatory style of dealing with patients appear to be the primary protection that physicians have against malpractice lawsuits. Patients are much less inclined to bring legal action against such physicians.

2.0.4 Psychological Significance of Patient Preferences: Control

Patient preferences are psychologically significant because the ability to express preferences and have others respect them is crucial to a sense of personal worth. The patient, already threatened by disease, may have a vital need for some sense of control. Furthermore, when patient preferences are ignored or devalued, patients are likely to distrust and perhaps disregard physicians' recommendations. When patients are overtly or covertly uncooperative, the effectiveness of therapy is threatened. Furthermore, patient preferences are important because their expression may lead to the discovery of other factors, such as fears, fantasies, or unusual beliefs, that the physician should consider in dealing with the patient.

2.0.5 Paternalism

A central ethical issue is the tension between autonomy and paternalism. The term "paternalism" refers to the practice of overriding or ignoring preferences of patients to benefit them or enhance their welfare. Ethically, paternalism represents the judgment that beneficence takes priority over autonomy. Historically, the medical profession endorsed paternalism; today, although still common, it is considered ethically suspect. Situations can occur, however, in which paternalistic behavior is ethically justified. These will be noted at various points in the subsequent pages.

Beauchamp TL, Childress JF. Paternalism: Conflicts between beneficence and autonomy. In: *Principles of Biomedical Ethics.* 5th ed. New York: Oxford University Press; 2001:176–191.

2.0 P The Preferences of the Child

As children become mature enough to articulate their preferences and reasons for them, they are entitled to increasing respect for these preferences. They are led toward responsible maturity by this respect and by education. However, it is sometimes difficult to decide how much respect to afford a child's preferences, especially when these seem to be contrary to the child's welfare. It is also difficult to discern how rational these preferences are because consequences, alternatives, and relative values are often not perceived clearly by young children. Ethical and legal standards for parental decisions are discussed at Sections 2.7 P and 4.1.2 P.

2.1 INFORMED CONSENT

Informed consent is the usual way in which patient preferences are expressed. Informed consent is the practical application of respect for the patient's autonomy. When a patient consults a physician for a suspected medical problem, the physician makes a diagnosis and recommends treatment. The physician explains these steps to the patient, giving the reason for the recommended treatment, the option of alternative treatments, and the benefits and burdens of all options. The patient understands the information, assesses the treatment choices, and expresses a preference for one of the options proposed by the physician. This ideal scenario captures the essence of the informed consent process. As an ethical basis for the patient-physician relationship, informed consent consists of an encounter characterized by mutual participation, good communication, mutual respect, and shared decision making. Informed consent should not designate a mechanical recitation of facts or a pro forma signature on a piece of paper. The phrase "I consented the patient," used by young clinicians to report that the patient had signed a consent form, reveals a fundamental misunderstanding of informed consent.

Informed consent requires a dialogue between physician and patient leading to agreement about the course of medical care. Informed consent establishes a reciprocal relationship or therapeutic alliance between physician and patient. After initial consent to treatment has occurred, a continuing dialogue between patient and physician, concerning the patient's continuing medical needs, reinforces the original consent. A properly negotiated informed consent benefits both the physician and the patient: a therapeutic alliance is forged in which the physician's work is facilitated because the patient has realistic expectations about results of the treatment, is prepared for possible complications, and is more likely to be a willing collaborator in the treatment. Despite a vast literature in law and ethics about the importance of informed consent, many studies reveal that physicians often fail to observe the practice and the spirit of informed consent.

Beauchamp TL, Childress JF. The meaning and justification of informed consent. In: *Principles of Biomedical Ethics.* 5th ed. New York: Oxford University Press; 2001:77–98.

Special Supplement: Empirical research on informed consent: An annotated bibliography. *Hastings Cent Rep* 1999;29(1):S1–S42.

Berg JW, Appelbaum PS, Lidz CW, et al. *Informed Consent: Legal Theory and Clinical Practice.* New York: Oxford University Press; 2001.

Katz J. *The Silent World of Doctor and Patient.* New York: The Free Press; 1984.

Case I. Mr. Cure, the patient with pneumococcal meningitis, is told that he needs immediate antibiotic therapy. After he is informed of the nature of his disease, the benefits and burdens of treatment, and the possible consequences of nontreatment, he expresses his preference by consenting to the antibiotic therapy. A therapeutic alliance that is clinically, ethically, and emotionally satisfactory is formed and reinforced when the patient recovers.

Case II. Mr. Cope is a 42-year-old man who was diagnosed as having insulin-dependent diabetes at the age of 18 years. Insulin was prescribed, and a dietary regimen recommended. In the intervening years, he has complied with his dietary and medical regimen but has experienced repeated episodes of ketoacidosis and hypoglycemia. His physician has regularly discussed with Mr. Cope the course of his disease and the treatment plan, and has inquired about his difficulties in coping with his condition. The physician proposes that Mr. Cope consider an implantable insulin pump that could improve glycemic control.

COMMENT. Case I exemplifies what might be called routine consent. The physician expresses clinical judgment by making recommendations to the patient regarding an appropriate course of care. The patient makes known his preference by consulting the physician for diagnosis and treatment and by accepting the physician's recommendations. Case II is also an example of routine consent, but it occurs in a chronic disease setting. Mr. Cope's doctor was assiduous in informing and educating his patient. Mr. Cope accepted the treatment regimen, and his compliance with it shows his preferences. He is now considering whether he will accept the benefits and risk of the insulin pump. However, in chronic diseases, which often have variable courses, the patient may not be fully informed about, or aware of, the future implications of treatment or nontreatment. We shall see problems develop in both these cases in the following pages.

2.1.1 Informed Consent: Definition and Standards

Informed consent is defined as the willing acceptance of a medical intervention by a patient after adequate disclosure by the physician of the nature of the intervention, its risks and benefits, and also its alternatives with their risks and benefits. How should the adequacy of disclosure of information by a physician be determined? One approach is to ask what a reasonable and prudent physician would tell a patient. This approach, which is the legal standard in some of the early informed consent cases, is increasingly being replaced by a new standard, namely, what information reasonable patients need to know to make rational decisions. The former standard affords greater discretion to the physician; the latter is more patient-centered. A third standard, sometimes called a "subjective" standard, is patient-specific. The question then is whether the information provided is specifically tailored to a particular patient's need for information and understanding. Although the law usually requires that the physician meet only the reasonable-patient standard, a physician who engages in a participatory style of shared decision making is likely to aspire to the requirements of a subjective standard. The reasonable-patient standard may be ethically sufficient, but the subjective standard is ethically ideal.

2.1.2 Scope of Disclosure

Many studies show that patients desire information from their physicians; many practitioners are aware that their patients appreciate information. In recent years, candid disclosure, even of "bad news," has become the norm. It is widely agreed that disclosure should include (1) the patient's current medical status, including the likely course if no treatment is provided; (2) the interventions that might improve prognosis, including a description and the risks and benefits of those procedures, and some estimation of probabilities and uncertainties associated with the interventions; (3) a professional opinion about alternatives open to the patient; and (4) a recommendation that is based on the physician's best clinical judgment.

In conveying this information, physicians should avoid technical terms, attempt to translate statistical data into everyday probabilities, ask whether the patient understands the information, and invite questions. Physicians are not obliged, as one court said, to give each patient "a mini-medical education." Still, physicians should strive to educate their patients about their specific medical needs and options.

2.1.3 Stringency

The moral and legal obligations of disclosure also vary with the situation; they become more stringent as the treatment situation moves from emergency through elective to experimental. In some emergency situations, very little information can be provided. Any attempt to inform may be at the price of precious time. Ethically and legally, information can be curtailed in emergencies (see Section 2.7.3). When treatment is elective, much more information should be provided. Finally, detailed and thorough information should accompany any invitation to participate in research, particularly if the research maneuver is not directed to the patient's therapy (see Section 4.7.5).

2.1.4 Comprehension

Discussions of informed consent usually emphasize the amount and kind of information the doctor provides. However, the comprehension of the patient is fully as important as the provision of the information. Some studies and many anecdotes suggest that comprehension by patients of medical information is not outstanding. At the same time, studies suggest that methods of communication are poor and that little effort is made to overcome barriers to comprehension. The physician has an ethical obligation to make reasonable efforts to ensure comprehension. Explanations should be given clearly and simply; questions should be asked to assess understanding. Written instructions or printed materials should be provided. Video or computer programs should be provided to guide patients who face complicated decisions, such as choosing between options for treatment of breast cancer or prostate cancer. Educational programs for patients with chronic disease should be arranged.

2.1.5 Documentation

The process of informed consent concludes with the patient's consent (or refusal). This consent is documented in a signed "consent form" that is entered in the patient's record. Health care institutions require signed documentation before a medical or surgical procedure is initiated. The document typically names the procedure and merely states that the risks and benefits have been explained to the patient. Although such a consent form may be legally appropriate, it hardly exemplifies an ethically appropriate process. The actual process and details of the consent interview should be documented in the medical record. The signed consent form is not a substitute for this more complete documentation, nor is it sufficient to demonstrate that informed consent has properly taken place.

2.1.6 Difficulties with Informed Consent

Many studies reveal that physicians consistently fail to conduct ethically and legally satisfactory consent negotiations. Physicians may be trapped in technical language, troubled by the uncertainty intrinsic to all medical information, worried about harming or alarming the patient, or hurried and pressed by multiple duties. In addition, patients may be limited in understanding, inattentive and distracted, or overcome by fear and anxiety. Selective hearing because of denial, fear, or preoccupation with illness may account for failure to comprehend what one might otherwise understand. Patients may believe that decisions are the physician's prerogative; physicians may not appreciate the rationale for the patient's participation.

Many physicians feel the informed consent requirement imposes an undesirable and perhaps impossible task: undesirable because adequately informing a patient takes too much time and might create unnecessary anxiety, and impossible because no medically uneducated and clinically inexperienced patient can truly grasp the significance of the information the physician must disclose. Even physicians, when they are patients, may not comprehend information germane to their own illness. For these reasons, physicians sometimes dismiss the informed consent requirement as a meaningless but bureaucratically necessary ritual. This is a sadly limited view of the ethical purpose of informed consent. Informed consent is not merely pushing information at a patient. It is an opportunity to initiate a dialogue between physicians and their patients in which both attempt to arrive at a mutually satisfactory course of action. Informed consent should result in shared decision making. The process, while difficult, is not impossible and is always open to improvement. The dialogue between physicians and patients is not only inhibited by limitations of physician communication and patient comprehension, it is limited by the inability of many physicians to listen carefully to their patients' words and the emotions underlying them. Finally, the time limits for patient visits imposed by some managed care plans and clinics, and reimbursement policies that compensate for procedures but not for education discouraging good communication.

2.2 DECISIONAL CAPACITY

Consent to treatment is complicated not only by the difficulties of disclosure but also by the fact that some patients lack the mental capacity to understand or to make choices. The law often uses the terms "competence" and "incompetence" to indicate whether persons have the legal authority to make personal choices, such as managing their finances or making health care decisions. Judges alone have the right to rule that a person is legally incompetent. Medical practitioners may encounter legally competent patients who appear to have their mental capacities compromised by illness, anxiety, pain, or hospitalization. We refer to this clinical situation as **decisional capacity or incapacity,** to distinguish it from the legal determination of competency. It is necessary to assess decisional capacity as an essential part of the informed consent process.

Beauchamp TL, Childress JF. Capacity for autonomous choice. In: *Principles of Biomedical Ethics.* 5th ed. New York: Oxford University Press; 2001:69–77.

Grisso T, Appelbaum. *Assessing Competence to Consent to Treatment.* Oxford University Press; 1998.

Special Section on Capacity, Decision Making and Informed Consent. *J Clin Ethics* 1998;9(3).

Carney MT, Neugroschl J, Morrison RS, et al. The development and piloting of a capacity assessment tool. *J Clin Ethics* 2001;12(1):17–23.

2.2.1 The Concept of Decisional Capacity

In a medical setting, a patient's capacity to consent to or refuse care requires at least an ability to understand relevant information, to appreciate the medical situation and its possible consequences, to communicate a choice, and to engage in rational deliberation about one's own values in relation to the physician's recommendations about treatment options. For patients who obviously possess the relevant abilities, the capacity to decide for themselves is not seriously questioned. Their right to make their own decisions on the basis of their preferences should be respected. Patients who clearly lack these abilities, for example, because they are unconscious or are manifestly disoriented and delusional, fall below the threshold of decisional capacity. For them a surrogate decision maker is required. It may be unclear whether certain patients are above or below the threshold for decisional capacity. These are the problematic ethical cases and may require judicial determination of competence or incompetence.

2.2.2 Determining Decisional Capacity

Decisional capacity refers to the specific acts of comprehending, evaluating, and choosing among realistic options. The first step in making a determination of capacity is to engage the patient in conversation, to observe the patient's behavior, and to talk with third parties—family, or friends, or staff. It is often difficult, however, to discern the signs of mental incapacity. For example, paranoid patients appear normal until certain questions trigger a delusional belief system. Patients who too quickly agree to a physician's recommendations may not really understand what is being proposed. The mental capacity of patients who refuse a low-risk, high-benefit treatment without which they face serious injury or death is naturally suspect.

Physicians, attempting to assess a patient's decisional capacity, should not depend on global descriptions such as schizophrenia, depression, or dementia. What is important is how these general psychologic states and psychiatric diagnoses affect the patient's ability to understand and choose in a particular situation. Many persons with mental disease retain the ability to make reasonable decisions about particular choices that face them.

When a clinician doubts a patient's decisional capacity to make particular choices, formal and informal tests for cognitive functioning, psychiatric disorders, or organic conditions that may affect decisional capacity can be used. However, no single test is sufficient to capture the complex concept of decisional capacity in a clinical setting. Some conditions, such as an affective state of anxiety or depression, may be transitory or reversible with psychiatric intervention. Other conditions, such as drug-induced confusion, may be resolved by titrating medication properly. But some problems, such as inability to understand simple explanations of facts, or fixed delusions, may be impossible to remedy. In cases where determination of capacity is problematic, clinicians should seek consultation from local resources, such as psychiatric liaison services, hospital risk managers, attorneys, ethics committees, or consultants. When clinical evidence is sufficient to show that a patient is decisionally incapacitated, an appropriate surrogate decision maker assumes authority, as explained in Section 2.7.

Case I. Mr. Cope, the 42-year-old man with insulin-dependent diabetes, is brought by his wife to the emergency department with complaints of a flulike syndrome with fever, myalgias, anorexia, vomiting, and gradually developing stupor. His wife reports that for 2 days, Mr. Cope has been unable to eat, drink, or take oral medications. On the day before he is examined, he also did not take his morning or evening insulin. On evaluation in the emergency department, he is stuporous but opens his eyes when people shout his name or pinch his skin. His vital signs are as follows: temperature, 39.1°C; BP, 100/70; and pulse, 110 and regular. Physical findings include prominent basilar rales in the right lung posteriorly and a cooler right foot in comparison with the left. The right femoral artery is palpable but diminished compared with the left; a bruit is noted over the right femoral; and no pulses are felt in the right leg distal to the femoral. Initial laboratory studies confirm the clinical impression of acute right lower-lobe pneumonia and diabetic ketoacidosis, and indicate the following serum chemistry levels: glucose, 754 mg/dL; sodium, 124 mEq/L; potassium, 5.6 mEq/L; chloride, 91 mEq/L; CO_2, 12 mEq/L; BUN, 60 mg/dL; and creatinine, 2.2 mg/dL. In addition, his arterial blood gas values are pH, 7.10; Po_2, 65 mm Hg; and Pco_2, 26 mm Hg. On the basis of these findings, the physicians proposed vigorous treatment for the diabetic ketoacidosis with IV insulin and fluid and electrolyte repletion. In addition, although the right lower-lobe pneumonia was thought to be viral, the physicians recommended antibiotics to cover the possibility of a community-acquired bacterial pneumonia or an aspiration pneumonia. Although Mr. Cope was generally somnolent and stuporous, he awoke while the IV was being inserted and stated loudly: "Leave me alone. No needles and no hospital. I'm OK." His wife urged the medical team to disregard the patient's statements, saying, "He is not himself."

COMMENT. We agree with Mrs. Cope's assessment of the situation. Mr. Cope has an acute crisis (ketoacidosis and pneumonia) superimposed on a chronic disease (type I diabetes) and he demonstrates progressive stupor during a 2-day period. At this time, he clearly lacks decisional capacity, although he could make decisions 2 days earlier before the onset of his illness, and he could possibly make his own decisions again when he recovers from the ketoacidosis, probably within the next 24 hours. At this moment, it would be unethical to be guided by the demands of a stuporous individual who lacks decision-making capacity. The cause of his mental incapacity is known and is reversible. Physicians and surrogate concur on the patient's incapacity and are agreed on the course of treatment in accordance with the patient's best interest. The physicians would be correct to be guided by the wishes of the patient's surrogate, his wife, and to treat Mr. Cope over his objections. Issues associated with surrogate decision making are discussed at Section 2.7. We shall encounter another problem with Mr. Cope at Section 2.5.

Case II. In the case presented at Sections 1.0.1 and 2.1, Mr. Cure has symptoms suggestive of bacterial meningitis. He is informed that he needs immediate hospitalization and administration of antibiotics. He refuses treatment and says he wants to go home. The physician explains the extreme dangers of going untreated and the minimal risks of treatment. The young man persists in his refusal. Apart from this strange demand, he exhibits no evidence of mental derangement or altered mental status.

COMMENT. There is no overt clinical evidence to support a judgment that Mr. Cure is incapacitated. The physician might presume altered mental status because of fever or metabolic disturbance, but mere presumption, in the absence of affective and behavioral clues, is inadequate to justify a conclusion that he is incapacitated. Physicians sometimes assume that any refusal of lifesaving treatment establishes incapacity, and they assume the person to be incompetent. Refusal of treatment should not, in and of itself, be considered proof of incapacity. Clinical evidence or solid medical reason must exist to justify the judgment of incapacity. Is it ethically permissible to treat against his will a patient with a life-threatening condition whose capacity to choose appears intact? The case is further discussed under enigmatic refusal (Section 2.5.2).

Case III. Mrs. D., aged 77 years, is brought to the emergency department by a neighbor. Her left foot is gangrenous. She has lived alone for the last 12 years and is known by neighbors and by her doctor to be intelligent and independent. Her mental abilities are relatively intact, but she is becoming quite forgetful and is sometimes confused. On her last two visits to her doctor, she consistently called him by the name of her former physician, who is now dead. On being told that the best medical option for her problem is amputation, she adamantly refuses, although she insists she is aware of the consequences and accepts them. She calmly tells her doctor (whom she again calls by the wrong name) that she wants to be buried whole. He considers whether to seek judicial authority to treat.

COMMENT. Mrs. D.'s mild dementia casts doubt on her ability to make an autonomous judgment. However, even persons whose mental performance is somewhat abnormal should not thereby be disqualified as decision makers. Persons might not be well oriented to time and place and still understand the issue confronting them. The central test of a person's competence is evidence that the nature of an issue and the consequences of any choice relating to the issue are understood. It is also possible to place any choice in the context of a person's own life history and values and ask whether the particular choice seems consistent with these. This is sometimes called the "authenticity" of the choice. Although ethicists argue over this as a criterion of mental capacity, it can often be a helpful clinical guide in evaluating the autonomy of the choice.

RECOMMENDATION. Mrs. D.'s clear assertions and the broader evidence of her life and values suggest that she has adequate decisional capacity to make an autonomous choice. Her physician should not seek a judicial determination of incompetence, unless genuine doubt exists about her decisional capacity. Treatment of Mrs. D. should be limited to appropriate medical management. It is appropriate to attempt gentle persuasion to accept amputation, but no undue pressure or coercion should be used.

Case III. (Continued). Mrs. D. comes to the emergency department as described previously. In this version of the case, however, she adamantly denies that she has any medical problem. Although the toes of her left foot are necrotic and gangrenous tissue extends above the ankle, she insists that she is in perfect health and has been taking her daily walk every day, even this morning. Her neighbor asserts that Mrs. D. has been housebound for at least a week, a fact that had led her to drop in to see whether there was a problem.

RECOMMENDATION. In this version, Mrs. D. seems decisionally incapacitated. She is denying her infirmity and her need for care and appears to be delusional. In Mrs. D.'s best interests (Sections 2.7.2 and 3.0.3), the appointment of a surrogate should be sought, and a decision about surgery considered.

2.2.3 Evaluating Decisional Capacity in Relation to the Need for Intervention

Usually a patient's capacity is not seriously questioned unless the patient decides to refuse or discontinue medically indicated treatment. In such situations, tests of capacity to consent might be applied. When patients reject recommended treatment, tests of capacity might be appropriate, because providers may suspect that the patients' choice may be harmful to their health and welfare. These tests can range from the simplest tests of mental status available to any physician to the more sophisticated evaluations applied by a psychiatrist or clinical psychologist. It has been suggested that the stringency of the test should vary with the seriousness of the disease and urgency for treatment; the standard of capacity required for decision making varies with the extent and probability of risk, with the extent and probability of benefit, and with consent or refusal. For example, a patient might need to meet a low standard of capacity to consent to a procedure with substantial, highly probable benefits and minimal, low-probability risk, such as antibiotics for bacterial meningitis. A higher standard of competence should be required to refuse the same treatment. Likewise, greater decisional capacity is necessary to consent to a high-risk, low-benefit intervention, such as stem cell transplantation for primary amyloidosis.

2.2.4 Waxing and Waning Capacity

Certain pathologic conditions, such as organic brain syndrome, are characterized by a movement in and out of mental clarity. Similarly, a patient's mental capacity often changes during the day, as in the so-called sundowner syndrome. Thus, a patient may at one time appear clear and oriented but later be assessed as incapacitated.

Example. Mrs. Care, with multiple sclerosis (MS), is now hospitalized. In the morning, she can converse intelligibly with doctors, nurses, and family. In the afternoon, she confabulates and is disoriented to place and time. In both conditions, she expresses various preferences about care that are sometimes contradictory. In particular, when questioned in the morning about surgical placement of a tube to prevent aspiration, she says no to the placement; in the afternoon, however, she speaks confusedly and repeatedly about having the tube placed.

RECOMMENDATION. This waxing and waning of mental status is itself the manifestation of disease. The patient should be considered to have impaired capacity. The expression of preferences in such a state should not be considered determinative, unless there is consistency in the preferences expressed during periods of clarity.

2.3 BELIEFS DUE TO RELIGIOUS AND CULTURAL DIVERSITY

Certain religious groups hold beliefs about health, sickness, and medical care that may be unfamiliar to providers. Sometimes such beliefs will influence the patient's preferences about care in ways that providers might consider imprudent or dangerous. Similarly, persons from cultural traditions differing from the prevailing culture may view the medical practices of the prevailing culture as strange and even repugnant. In both cases, providers will be faced with the problem of reconciling a clinical judgment that seems reasonable to them, and even an ethical judgment that seems obligatory, with a patient's preference for a different course of action. The appropriate response to such situations will be treated under the three topics where they usually appear: truthful disclosure (Section 2.4), competent refusal of treatment (Section 2.5), and the role of family in making decisions (Section 4.1.2, 4.1.2 P). Some general comments about appropriate responses are given in the following paragraphs.

(a) Unfamiliarity with beliefs and customs of others may lead providers to question the mental capacity of the patient. Physicians and nurses may suspect that anyone who refuses indicated treatment has impaired capacity. The mere fact of adherence to an unusual belief is not, in and of itself, evidence of incapacity. In the absence of clinical signs of incapacity, such persons should be considered capable of choice.

(b) In institutions where there is a high volume of patients from a particular religious or cultural tradition, providers must educate themselves about the beliefs of those patients, have competent translators available, and make use of mediators, such as clergy or educated persons who can explain the beliefs and communicate with those who hold them. At the same time, the mere fact that a person speaks the same language or comes from the same country or religion as the patient does not guarantee competence as a translator or intermediary. Also, providers should be careful to avoid cultural stereotypes: There are individuals from particular cultures who depart, in their values, preferences, and life style, from the predominant mode of their cultures.

(c) To the extent possible, a treatment course that is acceptable to the patient and provider alike should be negotiated. It is first necessary to discover the common goals that are sought by the patient and the physician and to settle on mutually acceptable strategies to attain those goals. The ethical response to a genuine conflict in an essential matter is dependent on the circumstances of the case and will be discussed below, under truthful communication and refusal of care. Cases in which cultural differences play a significant role are found in Sections 2.5.1, 2.7.5 P, and 4.5.

Special Section. Cross-cultural perspectives in health care. *Camb Q Healthcare Ethics* 1994;3(3).

Cultural differences in bioethics. *J Clin Ethics* 1993;4(2).

2.4 TRUTHFUL COMMUNICATION

Communications between physicians and patients should be truthful; that is, statements should be in accord with facts. If the facts are uncertain, that uncertainty should be acknowledged. Deception, by stating what is untrue or by omitting what is true, should be avoided. These ethical principles govern all human communication. However, in the communication between patients and physicians, certain ethical problems emerge about truthfulness. Does the patient really want to know the truth? What if the truth, once known, causes harm? Might not deception help by providing hope? In the past, medical ethics has given ambiguous answers to these questions: while some authors favored truthfulness, others recommended beneficent deception. More recently, with the prominence of the doctrine of informed consent, truthfulness has been commended as the ethical course of action.

Beauchamp TL, Childress JF. Veracity. In: *Principles of Biomedical Ethics.* 5th ed. New York: Oxford University Press; 2001;283–292.

Case I. Mr. R.S., a 65-year-old man, comes to his physician with complaints of weight loss and mild abdominal discomfort. The patient, whom the physician knows well, has just retired from a busy career and has made plans for a round-the-world tour with his wife. Studies reveal mild elevation in liver functions and a questionable mass in the tail of the pancreas. At the beginning of his interview with his physician to discuss the test results, Mr. R.S. remarks, "Doc, I hope you don't have any bad news for me. We've got big plans." Ordinarily, a needle biopsy of the pancreas to confirm pancreatic cancer would be the next step. The physician wonders whether he should put this off until Mr. R.S. returns from his trip. Should the physician's concern that Mr. R.S. may have pancreatic cancer be revealed to him at this time?

COMMENT. In recent years, commentators on this problem have moved away from the traditional medical ethics, which favored beneficent deception, toward a strong assertion of the patient's right to the truth. Their arguments are as follows:

1. There is a strong moral duty to tell the truth that is not easily overridden by speculation about the possible harms of knowing the truth.
2. Patients have a need for the truth if they are to make rational decisions about actions and plans for life.
3. Concealment of the truth is likely to undermine the patient-physician relationship. In case of serious illness, it is particularly important that this relationship be strong.

4. Toleration of concealment by the profession may undermine the trust that the public should have in the profession. Widespread belief that physicians are not truthful would create an atmosphere in which persons who fear being deceived would not seek needed care.

5. Suspicion on the part of the physician that truthful disclosure would be harmful to the patient may be founded on little or no evidence. It may arise more from the physician's own uneasiness at being a "bearer of bad news" than from the patient's inability to accept the information.

6. Recent studies have shown that most patients with diagnoses of serious illness wish to know the diagnosis. Similarly, recent studies are unable to document harmful effects of full disclosure.

7. The law has traditionally allowed physicians a so-called therapeutic privilege to withhold information under certain circumstances. However, those circumstances are very narrow. The California Supreme Court expressed it this way: "when a doctor can prove by a preponderance of the evidence he relied upon facts which would demonstrate to a reasonable man that the disclosure would have so seriously upset the patient that the patient would not have been able to dispassionately weigh the risks of refusing to undergo the recommended treatment." (*Cobbs v Grant,* 1972.)

In this strict interpretation, the therapeutic privilege is allowed only if the patient would be decisionally incapacitated by the knowledge.

RECOMMENDATION. Mr. R.S. should be told the truth: he probably has cancer of the pancreas. The considerations in favor of truthful disclosure are, in our opinion, conclusive in establishing a strong ethical obligation on the physician to tell the truth to patients about their diagnosis and its treatment. The following considerations are relevant:

(a) Speaking truthfully means relating the facts of the situation. This does not preclude a manner of relating the facts that is measured to perceptions of the hearer's emotional resilience and intellectual comprehension. The truth may be "brutal," but the telling of it should not be. A measured and sensitive disclosure is demanded by respect for the autonomy and the sensitivities of the patient. It reinforces the patient's ability to deliberate and choose; it does not overwhelm this ability.

(b) Truthful disclosure has implications for Mr. R.S.'s plans. Further diagnostic studies might be done and appropriate treatments chosen. The trip might be delayed or canceled. Estate planning might be considered. Mr. R.S. should have the opportunity to reflect on these matters and to take control of his future. If some facts have no implications for the patient's deliberation and choices, they need not be revealed.

Case II. Mr. S.P., a 55-year-old teacher, has had chest pains and several fainting spells during the past 3 months. He reluctantly visits a physician at his wife's urging. He is very nervous and anxious and says to the physician at the beginning of the interview that he abhors doctors and hospitals. On physical examination, he has classic signs of tight aortic stenosis, confirmed by echocardiogram. The physician wants to recommend cardiac catheterization and probably cardiac surgery. However, given his impression of this patient, he is worried that full disclosure of the risks of catheterization would lead the patient to refuse the procedure.

COMMENT. In this case, the anticipated harm is much more specific and dangerous than the harm contemplated in Case I. Hesitation about revealing the risks of a diagnostic or therapeutic procedure is based on the fear the patient will make a judgment detrimental to health and life. Also, in this case there is better reason to suspect this patient will react badly to the information than will the patient in Case I.

RECOMMENDATION. The arguments in favor of truthful disclosure apply equally to this case and to Case I. Whether or not catheterization is accepted, the patient will need further medical care. In fact, the situation is urgent. This patient needs, above all, the benefits of a good and trusting relationship with a competent physician. Honesty is more likely to create that relationship than deception. Also, the physician's fears about the patient's refusal may be exaggerated. In addition, studies indicate that almost all patients desire disclosure. The physician might also be concerned about the family's reaction if Mr. S.P. died unexpectedly during catheterization. Finally, the physician would be ethically and legally accountable for failing to advise the patient about the seriousness of his problem.

Case III. A person who tries to donate blood for a relative is found to be positive for HIV antibody. The blood is discarded and the donor's name registered as "deferred." Should the donor be informed?

RECOMMENDATION. The donor should be informed and counseled. Further confirmatory testing is necessary and advisable. Because a risk of infectivity exists, and it is possible that information about behavior may reduce that risk, the person has the right to this information and to education about HIV infection. In addition, treatment options for asymptomatic patients with HIV infection provide another reason to inform donors of their HIV status.

Case IV. A traditional Navajo man, 58 years old, is brought by his daughter to a community hospital that is authorized by the Indian Health Service to serve Native American patients. He is suffering severe angina. Studies show that he is a candidate for cardiac bypass surgery. The surgeon discusses the risks of surgery and says, as is his custom, that there is a slight risk that the patient may not wake up from surgery. The patient listens silently, returns home, and refuses to return to the hospital. His daughter, who is a trained nurse, explains: "The surgeon's words were very routine for him, but for my Dad it was like a death sentence."

Carrese JA, Rhodes LA. Western bioethics on the Navajo Reservation. *JAMA* 1995;274:826–829.

COMMENT. In Navajo culture, language has the power to shape reality. Thus, the explanation of possible risks is a prediction that the undesirable events are likely to occur. In that culture, persons are accustomed to speak always in positive ways and to avoid speaking about evil or harmful things. The usual practice of informed consent, which requires the disclosure of risks and adverse effects, can cause distress and drive patients away from needed care. Similar reservations about the frankness of informed consent are found in other cultures. This issue will be discussed again in Chapter 4, where we treat the role of the family (Section 4.1.2).

RECOMMENDATION. Physicians who understand this feature of Navajo life should shape their discussions in accordance with the expectations of the patient. The omission of negative information, even though it would be unethical in dealing with a non-Navajo patient, is appropriate. This ethical advice rests on the fundamental value that underlies the rule of informed consent, namely, respect for persons, which requires that persons be respected, not as abstract individuals, but as formed within the values of their cultures.

2.4.1 Completeness of Disclosure

Disclosure of options for treatment of a patient's condition should be complete, including the options that the physician recommends and also other options that the physician may believe are less desirable but which are still medically reasonable. In so doing, physicians may make it clear why they consider these other options less desirable. However, it might be asked whether the obligation of truthful disclosure requires telling a patient about even those interventions that are not medically reasonable, but which a patient may wish to consider.

Case I. A 41-year-old woman has a breast biopsy that reveals cancer. The physician knows that this patient has a history of noncompliance and cancellation of medical appointments. In light of this, the physician believes that the best treatment approach would be a modified radical mastectomy. Should he also describe an alternative approach that includes lumpectomy, breast reconstruction, and a 5-week course of radiation therapy? The physician is concerned that after a lumpectomy, the patient may not keep her appointments.

RECOMMENDATION. The entire range of options should be explained with a careful delineation of the risks and benefits of each. Making a strong argument in favor of the option the physician considers best is not ethically prohibited. Persuasion, however, should leave the patient free to choose, even if the physician believes she may choose the less effective option. Ultimately, the patient must make decisions about breast surgery and keeping appointments. The physician must provide the patient with information and encourage her to complete whatever form of treatment she elects to receive.

2.4.2 Disclosure of Medical Error

Medical errors occur frequently (Section 1.0.5). Some errors are due to negligence, but the majority are due to accident, misinformation, or organizational malfunction. Some errors do not cause harm; others effect serious harm. When medical errors occur, what obligations do physicians have to disclose them?

Case. The patient described in Section 2.4.1 is treated by modified radical mastectomy and reconstructive breast surgery. Postoperatively, she develops persistent swelling and drainage of the breast and a fever consistent with a breast abscess. She is returned to the operating room for exploration of the operative site. The surgeon discovers that a sponge had been left in the surgical wound; it is removed, and the abscess is treated. The patient recovered and was discharged. Should the physician inform the patient that a mistake had been made?

RECOMMENDATION. Disclosure is required because harm was done to this patient by the medical error. Although the outcome was satisfactory, the patient required a second operation with attendant risks; her hospital stay, with its attendant risks, was prolonged; and chemotherapy was delayed, and costs were incurred. Harms of this sort deserve apology, as a fundamental duty of respect for persons. The surgeon should inform the patient and the institution of the error, and appropriate compensatory measures should be taken.

COMMENT. The prevalent climate of secrecy about medical mistakes must be dispelled. Mistakes must be reported for risk management and quality assurance purposes, and organizations should have effective methods to do so. Organizations should also institute strong systems to prevent errors that might be due to system faults. Costs should be waived and appropriate compensation provided; settlement of financial claims, even without suit, may be considered. A climate of disclosure and honesty is necessary to maintain patient confidence and trust in the relationship with their physicians and with the health care institutions. Malpractice actions are certainly possible, particularly if the error is the result of negligence, but fear of legal claims is most probably misplaced if the context of confidence and honesty is sustained. Errors that are truly harmless, without any adverse effects for the patient, must be reported within the system for control purposes. Although it is not obligatory to disclose harmless error, it is advisable to do so to sustain the climate of honesty in the relationship between the patient and physician.

2.4.3 Placebos

Placebo is defined as a substance given in the form of medicine but lacking specific activity for the condition being treated. This must be distinguished from the "placebo effect," which is the psychologic, physiologic, or psychophysiologic effect of any medication given with therapeutic intent, but which is independent of any actual pharmacologic effects. The placebo effect is believed to occur as the result of many different influences: faith in the physician, administration of a medicine that the physician believes to be effective pharmacologically but is not, or actions of the physicians that are not in themselves therapeutic, such as taking a history or performing a diagnostic test. Thus, the placebo effect usually occurs without deliberate deception. In this broader sense, the placebo effect is a significant feature of medical practice, and the supposed benefits of a placebo treatment appear to depend on the qualities of the patient-physician relationship.

The problem of deception occurs when the physician knows that the intervention does not have the objective properties necessary for efficacy and when the patient is kept ignorant of this fact. Examples of such deception are monthly shots of vitamin B_{12} for fatigue without a diagnosis of pernicious anemia and penicillin administered for a viral sore throat. In some cases, the deception is an outright moral offense, motivated solely by the desire to keep the patient's fees or to "get the patient off my back"; in other cases, placebo deception may raise a genuine ethical question. The duty not to deceive seems to conflict with the duty to benefit without doing harm.

Placebo agents are now commonly used in controlled clinical trials of therapy for non-life-threatening conditions. Research subjects are informed that they will be randomized and may receive either an active drug or an inert substance. No deception is involved, and this practice is certainly ethical.

Beauchamp TL, Childress JF. Intentional nondisclosure. In: *Principles of Biomedical Ethics.* 5th ed. New York: Oxford University Press; 2001;83–88.

Case I. A 73-year-old widow lives with her son. He brings her to a physician because she has become extremely lethargic and often confused. The physician determines that, after being widowed 2 years before, she had difficulty sleeping, had been prescribed hypnotics, and she is now addicted. The physician determines the best course would be to withdraw her from her present medication by a trial on placebos.

Case II. A 62-year-old man has had a total proctocolectomy and ileostomy for colonic cancer. Evidence of any remaining tumor is absent; the wound is healing well, and the ileostomy is functioning. On the eighth day after surgery, he complains of crampy abdominal pain and requests medication. The physician first prescribes antispasmodic drugs, but the patient's complaints persist. The patient requests morphine, which had relieved his postoperative pain. The physician is reluctant to prescribe opiates because repeated studies suggest that the pain is psychologic, and the physician knows that opiates will cause constipation. She contemplates a trial of placebo.

COMMENT. Any situation in which placebo use involves deliberate deception should be viewed as ethically problematic. The strong moral obligations of truthfulness and honesty prohibit deception; the danger to the patient-physician relationship advises against it. In those situations, however, when deceptive placebo use seems indicated, its ethical use would require at least the following conditions: (1) The condition to be treated should be known as one that has high response rates to placebo, for example, mild mental depression or postoperative pain; (2) the alternative to placebo is either continued illness or the use of a drug with known toxicity, for example, hypnotics as in Case I or morphine in Case II; (3) the patient wishes to be treated and cured, if possible; and (4) the patient insists on a prescription.

RECOMMENDATION. The use of a placebo in Case I is not justified. The patient is not demanding medication. The problem of addiction should be confronted directly. There will be ample opportunity to develop a good relationship with this patient. Subsequent discovery of deception might undermine this relationship. Use of placebo in Case II is tempting but not ethically justifiable. In favor of placebo use, the patient is demanding relief. Morphine has adverse side effects. A short trial of placebo may be effective in relieving pain and avoiding the harm associated with opioids. However, explanation may be as effective as placebo use. The deceptive placebo can destroy the trust that creates the important and therapeutic "placebo effect" and can undermine the patient's confidence in the physician. A participatory style of decision making is based on honest communication. Consultation with the hospital pain service is recommended. Thus, even though we believe that placebo use might be theoretically justifiable, under the conditions expressed previously, use of placebos in practice is imprudent.

2.5 COMPETENT REFUSAL OF TREATMENT

Persons who are well-informed and have decisional capacity sometimes refuse recommended treatment. When the treatment is elective, ethical problems are unlikely. However, if care is judged necessary to save life or manage serious disease, physicians may be confronted with an ethical problem: Does the physician's responsibility to help the patient ever override the patient's freedom? Refusal of care by a competent and informed adult should be respected, even if that refusal would lead to serious harm to the individual. This is ethically supported by the principle of autonomy and legally supported by American law. The patient's refusal of well-founded recommendations is often difficult for the conscientious physician to accept. It is made more difficult when the patient's refusal, while competent, seems irrational, that is, deliberately contrary to the patient's own welfare.

Case I. Ms. T.O. is a 64-year-old surgical nurse. Five years ago she had a resection of a stage I infiltrating ductal carcinoma. She visited her physician again after discovering a 2-cm mass in the contralateral breast. Studies now reveal clinical stage II breast cancer with probable node involvement. The patient is informed of her condition and given options for treatment. She requests a lumpectomy with lymph node dissection. After surgery, 3 of 12 nodes are positive. Chemotherapy and radiation are recommended and Ms. T.O. is told that the statistics for her condition suggest that, with treatment, her long-term survival rate is about 60%. Without treatment, her disease-free survival rate is about 20%. She accepts chemotherapy, but after the first course, during which she has experienced significant toxicity, she informs her physician that she no longer wants any treatment. After extensive discussions with her physician and with her two daughters, she reaffirms her refusal of adjuvant therapy.

Case II. Mr. S.P., the patient with aortic stenosis described at Section 2.4, Case II, has cardiac symptoms that indicate the need for coronary angiography. On hearing his physician explain the urgency for this procedure and its benefits and risks, he decides he does not want it.

RECOMMENDATION. Ms. T.O. makes a competent refusal of treatment. She is well informed and she exhibits no evidence of any mental incapacitation. Even though the physician might consider the chances for prolonging disease-free survival good, Ms. T.O. values her risks and chances differently. Her refusal should be respected. The physician should continue to observe Ms. T.O., particularly for the next several months during which a change of mind in favor of adjuvant therapy would still be beneficial. In Case II, Mr. S.P. is also competent. His refusal, even though it seems contrary to his interests, from the point of view of his ability to anticipate his health needs, is an expression of his autonomy. It must be respected. That respect, however, also should encourage the physician to explore more fully the reasons for the refusal and to attempt to educate and persuade. An early follow-up visit should be scheduled for both patients to assure them that their physician remains supportive and concerned to help them deal with the consequences of their decision.

Case III. We have seen Mr. Cope (Section 2.2.2) admitted to the hospital for treatment of diabetic ketoacidosis with insulin, fluids, electrolytes, and antibiotics. That treatment was initiated over his objections but was authorized by his surrogate, Mrs. Cope, who was advised that his objections were the result of metabolic encephalopathy. After 21 hours, he awakens, talks appropriately with his family, and recognizes and greets his physician. He does not remember having been brought to the emergency department. He now complains to the nurse and physician about pain in his right foot and wonders whether the foot was injured inadvertently when he was unresponsive and brought to the emergency department. Examination of the foot reveals that it is cold and mottled in color compared with the left foot, and no pulses can be felt in the right leg distal to the right femoral artery. A vascular surgery consultation confirms by Doppler study that pulses distal to the femoral artery are absent and recommends an emergency arteriogram to determine whether the patient may have an embolic or thrombotic occlusion in the femoral system that may be treatable with angioplasty or embolectomy. This would prevent gangrene from developing in the right foot and leg and possibly prevent the need for amputation. After Mr. Cope is told the benefits and risks of the arteriogram, including the possible worsening of renal function, he declines to consent to arteriography. The surgeons explain to him that they cannot do angioplasty unless they know what vessel is involved and, in addition, they explain that it is very difficult, almost impossible, to perform exploratory vascular surgery without knowing in advance the site of the arterial occlusion. They warn the patient that he faces a greater risk of losing his leg than a risk of losing renal function. Mr. Cope participates in these discussions, asking appropriate questions, and acknowledging the doctors' comments. He then declines again to have the arteriography.

COMMENT. Although 24 hours ago, Mr. Cope was clearly decisionally incapacitated, and was properly treated for pneumonia and ketoacidosis, despite his insistence to be left alone, the current situation is entirely different. He has now regained decisional capacity, can understand the situation, can consider the risks and benefits, and make up his mind. His physician, nurses, and the consulting vascular surgeon agree that his decision is unwise: the low risk of worsening his renal function is more than compensated for by the substantial benefit of saving his leg. Mr. Cope does not agree. His family is divided, some siding with the doctors and some with Mr. Cope.

RECOMMENDATION. Mr. Cope's decision must be respected. Efforts can be made to persuade him otherwise; time can be given for reconsideration. Still, Mr. Cope shows no signs of incapacity and has the legal and moral right to make the decision that seems to him suitable. That decision may not be the best one from the viewpoint of medical indications, but law and ethics require respect for the patient's preferences in such circumstances.

2.5.1 Refusal on Grounds of Religious or Cultural Belief

We noted the problem of evaluating unfamiliar religious and cultural beliefs (Section 2.3). Persons who hold such beliefs sometimes refuse medical recommendations.

Case. Mr. G. comes to a physician for treatment of peptic ulcer. He says he is a Jehovah's Witness. He is a firm believer and knows his disease is one that may eventually require administration of blood. He quotes the biblical passage on which he bases his belief about blood transfusion not being used:

> "That ye abstain from meats offered to idols and from blood. . . .
> Acts 15:28.

The physician inquires of her Episcopal clergyman about the interpretation of this passage. He reports, after some research, that no

Christian denomination except the Jehovah's Witnesses takes this text to prohibit transfusion. The physician considers her patient's preferences impose an inferior standard of care. She wonders whether she should accept this patient under her care.

COMMENT. As a general principle, the unusual beliefs and choices of other persons should be tolerated if they pose no threat to other parties. The patient's preferences should be respected, even though they appear mistaken to others. The following general considerations apply to this case:

(a) Jehovah's Witnesses cannot be considered incapacitated to make choices unless there is clinical evidence of such incapacity. On the contrary, these persons are usually quite clear about their belief and its consequences. It is a prominent part of their faith, insistently taught and discussed. Thus, while others may consider it irrational, adherence to it is not, in itself, a sign of incompetence.

(b) Courts have almost unanimously upheld the legal right of adult Jehovah's Witnesses to refuse life-saving transfusions. If, however, unusual beliefs pose a threat to others, it is ethically permissible and may be obligatory to prevent harm by means commensurate with the imminence of the threat and the seriousness of the harm. Thus, courts have consistently intervened to order blood transfusions for the minor children of Jehovah's Witnesses. Courts were once inclined to order an adult transfused for the sake of the adult's minor children but will now rarely do so because alternative care for children is usually available.

(c) Refusal of blood transfusion differs in a significant way from refusal of all therapy or of recommended treatments. The Jehovah's Witnesses acknowledge the reality of their illness and desire to be cured or cared for; they simply reject one modality of care. Physicians may feel this limitation involves them in substandard and incompetent medical care.

(d) Refusal of transfusion may lead the physician to consider whether transfusion is necessary in this clinical situation. Some competent surgeons have undertaken to provide surgical procedures for Jehovah's Witnesses without the use of blood transfusion.

(e) The physician's inquiry about the interpretation of the biblical passage is interesting. Presumably, she would feel more comfortable with a belief she knew was endorsed by her own religious tradition. It is our opinion that the validity of a belief in an orthodox tradition is not relevant. Instead, the sincerity of those who hold it and their ability to understand its consequences for their lives are the relevant issues in this type of case.

RECOMMENDATION. Mr. G.'s refusal should be respected for the following reasons:

(a) If a Jehovah's Witness comes as a medical patient, as did Mr. G., the eventual possibility of the use of blood should be discussed and a clear agreement should be negotiated between physician and patient about an acceptable manner of treatment. It should be learned whether the patient rejects autologous transfusion, dialysis, and blood and blood products. Under no circumstances should the physician resort to deception. A physician who, in conscience, cannot accept being held to an inferior or dangerous standard of care should not enter into a patient-physician relationship or, if one already exists, should terminate it in the proper manner.

(b) If a Jehovah's Witness, who is known to be a confirmed believer, is in need of emergency care and refuses blood transfusion, the refusal ordinarily should be considered decisive. Even if the patient is mentally incapacitated at the time of the emergency, it can be presumed that the refusal represents the person's true wishes. However, if little is known about the patient and his or her status as a believer cannot be authenticated, treatment should be provided. In the face of uncertainty about personal preferences, it is our position that response to the patient's medical need should take ethical priority.

2.5.1 P Refusal of Treatment by Minor Children on Grounds of Religious Belief

Children may sometimes refuse medical treatment because they belong to religious groups that repudiate medical care. This poses a difficult problem for physicians.

Case I. James, a 14-year-old boy with acute lymphocytic leukemia, suffers his second relapse and fails to respond to chemotherapy. He is anemic and thrombocytopenic. He understands that transfusion would make him more comfortable, reduce the possibility of life-threatening bleeding, and perhaps allow him to leave the hospital. He affirms his belief as a Jehovah's Witness and refuses transfusion. His parents concur with his choice.

COMMENT. This boy is making an important decision: He is weighing his own discomfort against a belief about his eternal salvation. The medical value of the transfusion is, at best, limited. The boy is aware of his impending death and of the nature of his illness. He seems to show those characteristics of responsible decision making that we require in adults, even if we might suspect that, if more mature, he would see his beliefs differently. It is unethical to insist that he subordinate his beliefs for so transitory a benefit.

Case II. Karen, a 13-year-old, is sent from class to the school nurse complaining of severe headache and malaise. Noting her fever and irritability when moved, the nurse suspects meningitis. She calls the patient's mother, who says she will come directly to school. When the mother arrives, she informs the nurse that she and her husband are Christian Scientists. She says she will take Karen home where a Christian Scientist practitioner will pray for her. Karen's father soon arrives and reinforces the mother's position. They ask the nurse not to call a physician. When the nurse warns them about the extreme seriousness of Karen's condition, they remind her that Christian Scientist practitioners are considered health professionals under the law of their state. When the nurse asks Karen whether she wishes to be seen by a doctor, she affirms that she, too, believes in the doctrines of Christian Science and declines.

COMMENT. The consequences of refusing medical treatment for meningitis are very serious. Even if this youngster were not disoriented because of her illness, it is dubious that she would appreciate the dire consequences. Also, Karen's illness, unlike James's, is sudden and unexpected, and it is curable. Legally, her parents' refusal can be viewed as neglect and subject to the sanctions of state law. However, many states have enacted legislation exempting parents from charges of child abuse and neglect when they refuse medical interventions for religious reasons. Providers should be aware of the exact nature of these statutes and judicial decisions.

RECOMMENDATION. James's refusal of transfusions should be respected. Care should be directed to ensuring his comfort. Karen's refusal of medical care should not be accepted, and her parents' refusal should be opposed by providers, using the appropriate legal means. In general, the wishes of maturing children should be seriously considered in decisions about their care. Signs that the child has some comprehension of the situation and some appreciation of the consequences should be sought. Solicitous attention should be paid to helping them understand. The influences of fear and distress should be noted. Consultation with persons familiar with the psychology of the maturing child should be sought. Above all, nothing should be done to undermine the trust of the child in the adults who are responsible for care and upbringing.

2.5.2 Enigmatic Refusal

Occasionally, refusal of care may appear enigmatic: It is difficult to discern why a person should refuse an obvious benefit or to know whether they are really refusing.

Case. At Sections 2.1 and 2.2, Mr. Cure came to the emergency department with signs and symptoms suggestive of bacterial meningitis. When he was told his diagnosis and that he would be admitted to the hospital for treatment with antibiotics, he refused further care, without giving a reason. He would not engage in discussion with the staff about his refusal. The physician explained the extreme dangers of going untreated and the minimal risk of treatment. The young man persisted in his refusal and declined to discuss the matter further. Other than this strange adamancy, he exhibited no evidence of mental derangement or altered mental status that would suggest decisional incapacity.

COMMENT. In this case, the initial consent for diagnosis was implicit in the young man's coming to the emergency department. The patient's enigmatic refusal, however, unexpectedly introduced an incongruence between medical indications and patient preferences. It might be argued that the physician should simply permit the patient to refuse treatment and suffer the consequences, because the patient showed no objective signs of incapacitation or serious psychiatric impairment and because competent patients have the right to make their own (sometimes risky) decisions. However, when the risk of treatment is low and the benefit is great, the risk of nontreatment is high and the "benefits" of nontreatment are small, it is ethically obligatory for the physician to probe further to determine why the patient suddenly refused treatment. Despite explanation, has the patient failed to understand and appreciate the nature of the condition or the benefits and risks of treatment and nontreatment? If the patient seems to understand the explanation, is he denying that he is ill? Is the patient acting on the basis of some unexpressed fear, mistaken belief, or irrational desire? Through further discussion with the patient, some of these questions might be answered. Assume, however, that after the most thorough investigation possible under the urgent circumstances, evidence that the patient fails to understand is totally lacking, and nothing emerges to suggest denial, fear, mistake, or irrational belief. Should the patient's enigmatic refusal be respected? Because the medical condition is so serious, should treatment proceed even against the patient's will? This case poses a genuine ethical conflict between the patient's personal autonomy and the paternalistic values that favor medical intervention for the patient's own good. A clinical decision must be made quickly to treat or release the patient; good ethical reasons can be given for either alternative.

RECOMMENDATION. This patient's refusal is truly enigmatic. Evidence of an incapacity to choose because of an altered mental state is not present (although the patient's high fever and brain infection might lead the physician to suspect some derangement). In addition, the patient has not

expressed any religious objection to antibiotics. The patient simply refuses and will provide no reason for the refusal. Given both this enigmatic refusal and the urgent, serious need for treatment, the patient
should be treated, even against his will, if this is possible. Should there
be time, legal authorization should be sought. In offering this counsel,
we reluctantly favor paternalistic intervention at the expense of personal
autonomy. It is difficult to believe this young man wishes to die. The conscientious physician faces two evils: to honor a refusal that might not
represent the patient's true preferences, thus leading to the patient's serious disability or death, or to override the refusal in the hope that, subsequently, the patient will recognize the benefit. This is a genuine moral
dilemma: The principle of beneficence and the principle of autonomy
seem to dictate contradictory courses of action. In medical care, dilemmas cannot merely be contemplated; they must be resolved. Thus, we
resolve it in favor of treatment against the expressed preferences of this
patient.

In this case, we accept as ethically permissible the unauthorized
treatment of an apparently competent person. Recall that we endorsed
Mr. Cope's refusal of a useful therapeutic procedure (Section 2.5, Case
III). How do these apparently inconsistent recommendations differ? We
offer the following explanations:

(a) The medical indications are significantly different. Mr. Cure has a
critical disease, and low-risk antibiotic treatment will be effective in preventing serious harm. An opportunity is present for complete achievement of all medical goals. Mr. Cope is at risk of gangrene but is not now
critically ill.

(b) The consent situation is significantly different. In neither case is
there behavioral evidence of psychiatric impairment, yet in both, the
common psychologic mechanism of denial may hinder good judgment.
However, in the case of Mr. Cope, the refusal occurs after full disclosure
of his problem, the proposed procedure, and its risks. An opportunity for
discussion, persuasion, and argument has been presented. In Mr. Cure's
case, discussion is truncated. Efforts to discuss are rejected. Yet he has
willingly come to be treated. One might suspect that some crucial element of this negotiation is missing. It is this suspicion that leads the
physicians, given the medical situation, to treat him against his wishes.

(c) In fact, something was missing. Mr. Cure's brother had nearly died
10 years ago of an anaphylactic reaction to penicillin. But while in the
emergency department, Mr. Cure did not, and could not, recall this
event, and probing did not uncover it. Mention of antibiotics had trig-
gered a psychologic response of denial, which manifested itself in a refusal without reason. (The patient did not recall these events when re-

covered.) The circumstances of his particular illness drew the physicians in the direction of rapid treatment. Even though they made an effort to uncover the source of the problem, they failed to do so, and urgent need for treatment took priority.

(d) The case illustrates that physicians are often pressured by circumstances to make decisions before all relevant information is known. Thus, the rightness or wrongness of the clinical decision always must be assessed with respect to the clinician's knowledge at the time of the decision. We include this complex and troubling case to illustrate how actual situations do, at times, yield ambiguous results. One can only strive to render decisions that are as fully and carefully analyzed as the circumstances permit.

2.5.3 Refusal of Information

Persons have a right to information about themselves. Similarly, they have the right to refuse information or to ask the physician not to inform them.

Case I. Mr. A.J. is scheduled for surgery for spinal stenosis. The neurosurgeon begins to discuss the risks and benefits of this surgery. The patient responds, "Doc, I don't want to hear anything more. I want the surgery. I realize there are risks, and I have confidence in you." The surgeon is concerned that he has not completed an adequate disclosure.

Case II. Mrs. Care, with MS, had shown little interest during the early years of her illness in learning about the possible course of her disease. She refused frequent offers by the physician to discuss it. However, on one of her repeated admissions for treatment of urinary tract infection, she states that, had she known what life would be like, she would have refused permission for treatment of other life-threatening problems. The patient's mental status is difficult to evaluate; some clinicians think she shows signs of early dementia. Should she have been informed of her prognosis at an earlier time even though unwilling to engage in such discussions with her physician?

COMMENT. We are concerned with what the physician communicates and should communicate about diagnosis and, particularly, prognosis. Should the physician override the patient's stated preference not to know about her condition? Should physicians withhold unpleasant information about prognosis to protect the patient from depression or other negative, potentially damaging emotions? Or should the patient be told enough to maximize her opportunity to plan her life in the face of future prospects? Although it is tempting to withhold information to protect the patient, a better alternative would be to give the patient general information sufficient to indicate the seriousness of her condition as well as the uncertainty about the time, the severity, and the extent of the problems that MS can cause. This avoids the extremes of withholding too much too long or disclosing too much too soon. Considerable tact is required to find the proper balance of disclosure and reticence. Furthermore, the disclosures made as the condition worsens must be adjusted in the light of the impairments to the patient's capacity. In some cases of late-stage MS an associated dementia appears. Thus, it would be advisable to make disclosures before the patient's capacity is so severely impaired that she cannot understand.

RECOMMENDATION. In Case I, Mr. A.J.'s refusal of information should be respected. His surgeon need not continue the discussion but must make a full notation in the chart that the patient has refused information. It may be desirable to seek the patient's permission to discuss the detail of the procedure with an involved family member. Case II poses a difficult case in which unpleasant but unavoidable moral choices must be made. Here we opt for more rather than less disclosure, because the condition, though untreatable, is long-lasting. Thus, the patient's long-term autonomy is respected more by providing as much information as possible to enable her to make more choices while she is physically and mentally able to learn coping mechanisms in advance. The short-term gains of ignorance are outweighed by the long-term benefits of knowledge.

2.6 ADVANCE PLANNING

Persons are frequently concerned that when crucial decisions must be made about their medical care, they will no longer be capable of participating in those decisions. It is essential that they discuss these concerns with their family and their health care providers; it is also essential that physicians foster such discussions and record them in the patient's record. In recent years, the concept of advance planning has emerged and been widely promoted as a solution to that problem. The general term "advance planning" covers (1) the legal instrument entitled "Directive to Physicians" in the natural death acts enacted by various states, (2) the less formal "living will", and (3) the "durable (or medical) power of attorney for health care." Each of these forms is explained in the following paragraphs.

Advance directives of some kind have legal validity in every state. Most people agree, at least in principle, with the idea that individuals should be permitted to express their preferences concerning terminating or continuing life support in a legally effective document. In 1990, the

United States Supreme Court stated that persons have a constitutionally protected "liberty interest" in refusing unwanted medical treatment; this interest is not extinguished after mental capacity is lost. At the same time, the Court upheld a Missouri statute requiring "clear and convincing evidence" of an incapacitated person's prior wishes (*Cruzan v Missouri Dept. of Health,* 1990).

The idea of advance directives has become both familiar and accepted in ethics and in law. Medicare regulations require hospitals to provide patients with information about their rights under local law to accept or refuse recommended care and to formulate advance directives. In 1990, Congress passed the Patient Self-Determination Act requiring that all hospitals receiving federal funds, such as Medicare and Medicaid payments, must ask patients at the time of admission whether they have advance directives. If they do, patients are asked to submit copies for their records; if they do not, they are to be informed that they have the right to sign such a document and be given information about it. Advance directives have become more common in routine medical care and especially important in terminal care. In light of these developments, physicians should become familiar with the provisions of advance directives that are legally valid in their locale. Physicians should know the differences between the three principal forms of advance directives: natural death acts, durable power of attorney for health care, and living wills.

Although the legality of advance planning has been formalized by legislation and upheld by courts, medical practice has been slow to respond to the preferences of terminally ill patients for less aggressive end-of-life care. Several empirical studies document that physicians are reluctant to discuss end-of-life issues with patients known to be dying. Physicians often failed to write DNAR orders for patients who had requested them to do so. Systematic attempts to improve communication, information, and conversation between patients and physicians met with little success. Nor did the use of outcome data or patient preferences influence physician practices. End-of-life care, at least in the intensive care setting, is currently driven more by traditional hospital and physician practices to prolong life than by patient preferences.

SUPPORT Principal Investigators. A controlled trial to improve care for seriously ill hospitalized patients. *JAMA* 1995;274:1591–1598.

The SUPPORT Project: Lessons for action. *Hastings Cent Rep* 1995;25(6):S21–S22.

Beauchamp TL, Childress JF. Protecting incompetent patients. In: *Principles of Biomedical Ethics.* 5th ed. New York: Oxford University Press; 2001:152–157.

Special Supplement on Advance Care Planning. *Hastings Cent Rep* 1994; 24(6):S32–S36.

2.6.1 Types of Advance Directives

Several different types of advance directives are presently in use. Although different in form and legal implications, all should be taken as evidence of a patient's preferences. These various types are discussed in the following paragraphs.

Natural Death Acts. These are statutes passed by state legislatures. These statutes affirm a person's right to make decisions regarding terminal care and provide directions about how that right can be effected after the loss of decision-making capacity. Typically, they contain a model (or sometimes mandatory) document, called **Directive to Physicians.** These directives, which a patient can sign and give to the physician, are typically worded in this fashion: "If at any time I should have an incurable injury, disease, or illness certified to be a terminal condition by two physicians, and where the application of life-sustaining procedures would serve only to artificially prolong the moment of my death, and where my physician determines that my death is imminent whether or not life-sustaining procedures are used, I direct that such procedures be withheld or withdrawn, and that I be permitted to die naturally." Various natural death acts contain specific provisions concerning a variety of topics. The topics include personalized instructions, proxy appointments, whether a declaration is part of one's medical record, an immunity clause for physicians who carry out patient directives, terminal condition diagnosis, witness requirements, and permission or prohibition of withdrawing or withholding of ventilators, dialysis, artificial feeding, hydration, and so forth. Clinicians should know the specific features of the natural death acts of their states.

Living Wills. Advance directives may be communicated by a person to physicians, family, and friends in less formal, less legalistic fashion. One widely used model document contains the following words:

> "If I become unable, by reason of physical or mental incapacity, to make decisions about my medical care, let this document provide the guidance and authority needed to make any and all such decisions. If I am permanently unconscious or there is no reasonable expectation of my recovery from a seriously incapacitating or lethal illness or condition, I do not wish to be kept alive by artificial means."

"A Christian Affirmation of Life: A Statement on Terminal Illness," designed by the Catholic Health Association, contains the following words:

> "I have a right to make my own decisions concerning treatment that might unduly prolong the dying process. If I become unable to make these decisions and have no reasonable expectation of recovery, then

> I request that no ethically extraordinary means be used to prolong my life but that my pain be alleviated if it becomes unbearable."

Other versions have been proposed. Individuals may choose to compose their own form of the living will. In some states, these personal documents are given legal standing equivalent to a statutory **Directive to Physicians**. Even if there is no explicit legal recognition of personal documents, physicians should take account of them as expressions of their patient's preferences.

Choice in Dying. A Good Death: Taking More Control at the End of Your Life. Reading, Mass: Addison-Wesley; 1992.

A Christian Affirmation of Life. St. Louis: Catholic Hospital Association; 1974.

2.6.2 The Durable Power of Attorney for Health Care

State legislatures may pass a statute authorizing what is called "a durable power of attorney." These statutes authorizes individuals to appoint another person, called an "attorney-in-fact" (who need not be an "attorney-at-law"), to act as their agent to make all health care decisions after they have become incapacitated. This person may be a relative or friend. Most statutes require that this appointment be made in writing, although at least one state (California) permits oral designation of the attorney-in-fact. These statutes are particularly useful to physicians and hospitals because they authorize a specific decision maker, chosen by the patient, to make medical decisions on the patient's behalf. These statutes give legal priority to the attorney-in-fact over all other parties, including next of kin. This clarifies the confusion that often exists about who in the family is the appropriate decision maker for an incapacitated relative. It also avoids the bureaucratic burdens and costs of a legal proceeding to appoint a guardian or conservator.

2.6.3 Interpretation of Advance Directives

Written advance directives are an important innovation in the expression of patient preferences. They allow persons to project their preferences into the future for consideration by those responsible for their care when they themselves are incapable of expressing preferences. Advance directives do, however, present some problems to those to whom they are addressed. As written documents, they employ terms that are vague, such as "if there is no reasonable expectation of recovery" or the direction to forgo "artificial means and heroic measures." Such language requires interpretation in the setting of the case. In addition, they usually do not specifically indicate which of the various means of life-sustaining treatments the patient would wish forgone. Finally, some commentators wonder whether preferences expressed while a person enjoys decisional capacity should be honored after the patient has permanently lost such capacity and their personality has radically changed. Thus, although these documents are helpful as evidence about the patient's prior preferences and should be taken seriously, they do not replace thoughtful and responsible interpretation in the particular case.

Case I. Mrs. Care, with MS, is now hospitalized because of aspiration pneumonia. She is alternatively obtunded and severely confused. She had given her physician a copy of the Directive to Physicians 2 years earlier. Now, in reviewing the directive, the physician notices the words (common in these documents), "the patient's death must be imminent, that is, death should be expected whether or not treatment is provided." Should the physician consider that if intubation is medically indicated, it should be withheld in accord with the patient's prior preferences?

Case II. Mrs. A.T., a 70-year-old woman, very active and in good health, suffers a stroke after finishing a game of golf. She is admitted to the hospital unconscious and in respiratory distress. Studies show a brainstem and cerebellar infarct with significant edema involving the brainstem. She is provided ventilatory support. Her sister brings to the hospital a recently signed and witnessed Living Will. It contains the words, "I fear death less than the indignity of dependence and deterioration." The patient is currently unable to communicate. She is intubated and has cardiac arrhythmias. The neurologist believes that this patient has a good chance of recovery with little functional deficit; he mentions to the sister that she might have some gait disturbance. The sister responds, "I know she wouldn't want to live with that." Should her physician, on becoming aware of the living will, extubate her? Should no-code orders be written?

Case III. Mr W.W., a brilliant academic, appointed his wife medical attorney-in-fact with instructions not to provide artificial nutrition or hydration if he became severely demented. Mr. W.W. is now demented but maintains a pleasant affect, though he cannot converse and no longer recognizes family. He is now unable to feed himself or take food by mouth. The nursing home proposes to place a percutaneous endoscopic gastrostomy (PEG) tube to provide nutrition and hydration. His wife refuses to allow this; the nursing home administrator argues that Mr. W.W. is no longer the person who executed the advance directive but a "pleasantly demented individual" who may be enjoying his life.

RECOMMENDATION. In Case I, the physician may withhold intubation on the basis of the patient's advance directive. The words "whether or not treatment is provided" are a clumsy attempt to define the imminence of death. In this case, those words should not obstruct the fulfillment of Mrs. Care's preferences, which seem quite clear. In Case II, withdrawing ventilatory support is premature given the facts of the case. It is as yet unclear whether Mrs. A.T. will suffer "the indignity of dependence and deterioration." However, if the patient's condition deteriorates, it may be appropriate to reconsider this opinion. At this point, a DNAR order is also premature. However, if she recovers her ability to communicate and is competent, the exact meaning of her living will should be explored with her. In Case III, we believe Mr. W.W.'s instructions should be respected even in his present state, because when he had the capacity, he obviously considered situations just such as this. We believe that choices made on the basis of stable values should be honored.

2.7 DECISION MAKING FOR THE MENTALLY INCAPACITATED PATIENT

Persons receiving medical care occasionally cannot make decisions in their own behalf. They can neither give consent to treatment nor refuse it. Their incapacity may have many causes. They may be unconscious or uncommunicative or both. They may be suffering from mental disabilities, either transitory, such as confusion or obtundation, or chronic, such as dementia or a mental disease of some sort. When this occurs, decisions about the proper care of these persons must be made. Questions then arise, such as "Who is the suitable decision maker and what are the principles that should govern such decisions?"

Beauchamp TL, Childress JF. A framework of standards for surrogate decision making. In: *Principles of Biomedical Ethics.* 5th ed. New York: Oxford University Press; 2001:98–103.

Beauchamp TL, Childress JF. Protecting incompetent patients. In: *Principles of Biomedical Ethics.* 5th ed. New York: Oxford University Press; 2001:152–157.

Buchanan AE, Brock DW. *Deciding for Others: The Ethics of Surrogate Decision Making.* Cambridge: Cambridge University Press;1989.

Special Section: Substituted Judgment. *J Clin Ethics* 1995;6(1).

Special Section: When Others Decide. *Camb Q Healthcare Ethics* 1999;8(2).

2.7.1 Surrogate Decision Makers

A person who is authorized to make a decision on behalf of another who is incapacitated is called a **surrogate** or a **proxy.** Traditionally, next of kin have been considered the natural surrogates, and medical providers have turned to family members for their consent. This practice appears to have been tacitly accepted in Anglo-American law, but until recently was rarely expressed in statutes. In recent years, many states have enacted legislation that gives specific authority to family members and ranks them in priority (for example, spouse, parents, children, siblings). The durable power of attorney statutes also provide for a surrogate, given the technical title "attorney-in-fact," who supersedes family members. These statutes avoid the need to seek judicial recourse, except in cases of conflict or doubt about legitimate decision makers. Finally, all states have provisions for the judicial appointment of guardians or conservators for those declared incompetent by a judge.

2.7.2 The Principle of Surrogacy

When someone is granted authority to decide on behalf of the patient, that person's decisions must promote the patient's preferences and welfare.

When the patient's preferences are known, the surrogate must use knowledge of these preferences in making medical decisions. This is called the "substituted judgment" standard, and is used in two situations: (1) where the patient has previously expressed her preferences, and (2) where the guardian can reasonably infer the patient's preferences from past statements or actions. In either case, the surrogate decision maker must use knowledge of these preferences in making medical decisions for the incompetent patient.

The first situation is the most straightforward case, ethically speaking, and occurs when the patient has previously expressed preferences concerning the course of action she would desire in the present circumstances. Whether the patient recorded these preferences in writing or merely informed another person of the preferences orally, the surrogate should follow the patient's preferences as closely as possible. In effect, the surrogate is not making medical decisions for the patient, but is merely giving effect to decisions the patient made for herself. Courts typically apply this standard in situations where the patient's preferences are known. In a landmark case, In the Matter of Karen Quinlan (1976), the New Jersey Supreme Court was faced with the difficult decision of whether to permit the withdrawal of a respirator from a young woman in a persistent vegetative state with no chance for recovery. Before the accident that led to her impaired condition, the patient had made statements indicating that she would not want to be kept alive by extraordinary means if there was little chance for recovery. The court relied on these statements in applying the substituted judgment standard to order the removal of the respirator.

A more difficult decision occurs when the patient has not specifically stated what she would want, given the present circumstances. In such a case, a surrogate should use knowledge of the patient's values and beliefs in making a decision for the patient Surrogates must be careful to avoid the common ethical pitfall of injecting their own values and beliefs into the decision-making process, as only the patient's values and beliefs are relevant to the decision. Only individuals with a close association to the patient should attempt to act as a surrogate in situations where the patient's specific preferences are unknown but may be inferred from the patient's past actions and statements. In the well-known Cruzan case, the United States Supreme Court was confronted with a request to remove artificial nutrition and hydration tubes from a young woman in a coma. The patient had previously made statements to her roommate that she would not want to continue her life if she could not live "halfway normally." The Court, while endorsing the substituted judgment standard, declined to order the removal of the tubes, because the evidence about the patient's preferences failed to meet Missouri's evidentiary standards. The Court ruled that each state can adopt its own evidentiary standards in such cases.

Studies have shown that surrogates often mistakenly believe that they know what their family member would have wanted. Still, legitimate surrogates must be permitted to make these decisions as long as clinicians believe they are acting in good faith.

If the patient's own preferences are unknown or are unclear, the surrogate must consider the **best interests of** the patient. This requires that the surrogate's decision must promote the individual's welfare, which is defined as making those choices about relief of suffering, preservation or restoration of function, and the extent and sustained quality of life that reasonable persons in similar circumstances would be likely to choose. The concept of best interest is discussed at Section 3.0.3.

2.7.3 Implied Consent

In life-threatening emergencies, patients may be unable to express their preferences or give their consent because they are unconscious or in shock. No surrogate may be available. In such situations, it has become customary for physicians to presume that the patient would give consent if able to do so, because the alternative would be death or severe disability. This is a reasonable presumption. The law has accepted it under the somewhat inaccurate title of "implied consent." This is a legal fiction, because the patient is not actually consenting; the physician is presuming consent. Nonetheless, although a physician does not have any authority to extend treatment beyond the areas to which the patient has consented, the physician may presume consent when immediate action is necessary to preserve the patient's life. This provides the physician with a defense against a subsequent charge of battery (although it may not defend against charges of negligence if the emergency treatment falls below acceptable standards of care). From the ethical point of view, the principle of beneficence, which prescribes that a person has a duty to assist someone in serious need of help, is the ethical justification for emergency treatment of the incapacitated person.

2.7.4 Statutory Authority to Treat

In all jurisdictions, statutes exist that authorize psychiatrists to hold certain persons for psychiatric treatment against their will. These statutes pertain to persons who are suffering from mental disease, and the treatment authorized is treatment for mental disease. In addition, the person must be considered a danger to self or others. In some situations, both mental disease and medical problems may be present.

Case. A middle-aged man, known to the emergency department staff as psychotic and alcoholic, is brought to the hospital by a friend. He has been drinking and using heroin, and is hallucinating that Viet Cong are attacking him. He is breathless, has fainted twice in the last hour, and is incontinent of urine. He says his heart is breaking through his chest. Still, he says he must leave the hospital because it is being bombed. The admitting resident writes in the chart, "I noted hallucinations and psychotic ideation; thus, I am putting the patient on a medical hold and keeping him in the hospital for observation. Diagnosis: paroxysmal supraventricular tachycardia. Medications: haloperidol, digitalis. Further evaluation: assess electrolytes."

COMMENT. The question is whether the statutory authorization for involuntary hospitalization for psychiatric evaluation and treatment, sometimes inappropriately called a "medical hold," allows both medical treatment and treatment for mental illness. The answer is it does not. The statutes refer to the treatment of mental illness alone as the justification for involuntary commitment. If medical treatment is needed, the patient must consent or, if unable to do so, a legally authorized decision maker must be appointed. If medical treatment is needed for a life-saving emergency, implied consent suffices.

RECOMMENDATION. A number of mistakes were made in this case. First, the emergency department resident should have immediately sought psychiatric consultation. The consulting psychiatrist will examine the patient and, having made a diagnosis of paranoid schizophrenia, may authorize involuntary commitment for treatment of this mental disorder.

The ED resident does not have this authority. The term "medical hold" is misleading for two reasons: Physicians, other than psychiatrists, cannot "hold" patients, and the treatments offered are only psychiatric.

2.7 P Authority of Parents

Children, whose mental capacities mature as they develop, are considered incompetent under the law. The medical care of infants and children is authorized by the usual surrogates, namely the parents of the child, or in unusual circumstances, by other parties authorized by law. In addition, the law designates the age at which young persons are deemed capable of consent. Two ethical issues appear: First, it is sometimes necessary to determine the relevance and weight of parental preferences when these preferences conflict with the recommendations of providers. Second, children become capable of expressing their preferences at various ages. When they do express preferences, it is necessary to determine how reasonable and relevant these preferences are in matters of medical care.

Parental responsibility is a moral, social, and legal matter. It is commonly agreed that parents have the responsibility for the well-being of their children and that they have a wide range of discretion to determine the particular circumstances that this well-being will encompass. At the same time, parental discretion is not absolute. Infants and children are, in American law, considered persons, with certain interests and rights that must be acknowledged regardless of their parents' preferences. Thus, it is usually said that the best interests of the child set limits on the discretion of parents about the medical treatment of their offspring. Also, American society accepts, as an obligation, the protection of children from harm, even at the hands of their parents. Further, the welfare of children is taken as a serious social obligation.

2.7.1 P Determination of Parental Responsibility

In our society, biological parents may have various sorts of moral relationships to their offspring. Most parents eagerly and willingly accept their responsibility to nurture and educate their children. Some parents have conceived unwillingly and desire to be rid of their offspring before or immediately after birth. Others, because of various attitudes or disorders, have no concern for the child they have borne. Other parties, such as adoptive parents, assume certain responsibilities, perhaps even before legally authorized. Because of shifting social relationships, various adults may undertake moral or legal care of the child at different times. Even if it is possible to determine who bears legal authority, it is not always easy to see who has moral responsibility. Thus, while biological and social parents are the natural surrogates for children, in certain circumstances they may be incapable or incompetent to perform that responsibility. In American law, parents have fundamental rights over the care of their children that do not evaporate because they are not model parents. Still, it is clear in the law that the well-being of the child takes precedence over the parents' rights.

2.7.2 P Parental Incapacity

Pediatricians and other providers may occasionally suspect parents of serious incompetence in the care of their child. This suspicion must be cautiously evaluated. In some cases, a parent or parents may manifest the signs of a psychiatric disorder that might render them incapacitated for rational consideration of matters concerning their child. A psychiatrically disabled parent may constitute a danger to the child. The existence and extent of psychiatric disease should be evaluated and, if indicated, legal steps should be taken to provide a surrogate decision maker. Another sort of incompetence is manifested by parents who seem unable to comprehend the needs and interests of a child. Incompetence of this sort is most clearly manifest by overt and habitual physical abuse of a child. Failure to provide for the ordinary needs of a child may represent incompetence caused by ignorance, moral turpitude, or substance addiction. In other cases, failure may be due to parental inexperience or to social conditions. Suspicion of incompetence should be evaluated for its degree, causes, remediability, and so forth. Most important, the alleged incompetence should be relevant to the problem at hand. Social workers and others expert at evaluation of social and environmental conditions are invaluable contributors. If suspicions are verified, legal remedies may be sought depending on the seriousness and urgency of the situation. Child protective services exist in every jurisdiction to assist, if this step is necessary.

2.7.3 P Standard for Parental Preferences

When parents are properly identified and appear competent as decision makers, they are morally and legally required to observe certain standards in their decision for their child. The federal Baby Doe Rules state as follows:

> "The decision to provide or withhold medically indicated treatment is, except in highly unusual circumstances, made by the parent or legal guardians. Parents are the decision makers concerning care for their disabled infant, based on the advice and reasonable medical

judgment of their physician . . . this role must be respected and supported unless they choose a course of action inconsistent with the applicable standards established by law." (50 Code of Federal Regulations, at 14880.)

And, it may be added, inconsistent with moral principle. What standards, then, must guide parental choice? We offer the following considerations:

(a) It is clear that medical inefficacy or futility justifies a parental decision to discontinue treatment (Section 1.2 P). However, physicians and parents may disagree about the presence of these conditions. Parents may see as inefficacy the failure of a treatment to produce an immediate result or, overcome by the frustration of a long illness, conclude that treatment is futile. The physician has the duty to educate the parents, to explain the medical situation, and to strive to achieve a common understanding. Naturally, every effort must be made to reach an amicable understanding. However, it must be clear that the physicians and the institution have no ethical obligation to continue to provide treatment that, in their best professional judgment, is inefficacious or futile. In extreme cases, legal steps might be taken to relieve the institution of responsibility.

(b) It is equally true that physicians may be deluded by their own uncertainty, fear, or therapeutic or scientific zeal, and thereby fail to recognize or admit that current or proposed interventions are ineffective or are futile. This attitude, which can lead to ethical disasters, can be countered by rigorous honesty, genuine humility, and the willingness to listen to the opinions of others.

(c) Every pediatrician recognizes that the birth of a defective infant or the critical illness of a child can be a most traumatic experience for parents. Even the most lucid explanations of the medical problem can be misunderstood. It is difficult for parents to be properly informed and fully consenting surrogates. Nevertheless, it is also wrong to disqualify all parents as decision makers on the supposition that no one can make good decisions in a crisis. Each case must be judged on its own. Serious efforts at psychologically and emotionally suitable communication must be made.

(d) If intervention is not clearly ineffective or futile, decisions should be made in view of the best interests of the infant or child. The phrase "best interests" is explained at Sections 2.7.2, 3.0.3, and 3.0.1 P. Here the interests of the decision makers, namely, the parents and the physicians, or the interests of society at large are not the central focus: The interests of the patient constitute the standard for decisions made by others on behalf of that patient.

(e) A parental refusal of a recommended medical intervention should be respected unless the failure to provide the intervention would be likely to cause direct and serious harm to the child. Thus, a refusal to have a child immunized, although misguided, should be respected (unless it violates a statutory law) because it is impossible to demonstrate that an unimmunized child will be infected.

(f) In cases where differences of opinion exist between parents and physicians or between parents themselves, a review by an ethics committee or an ethics consultation may be helpful. If differences are irreconcilable, it may be necessary to have recourse to the legal system that has been established to protect the welfare of those incapable of protecting themselves. Such recourse is often extremely traumatic for all concerned, but it acknowledges that the infant or child, despite its inability to speak for itself, has a valued place in our society.

2.7.4 P Legal Consent of Minors

Minors, that is, persons who are younger than the statutory age of consent (18 years in all states), may come to a physician on their own initiative. When their medical problem is not an emergency, such persons can be treated only with the consent of their parents or legal guardian (Section 2.7 P). However, there are several exceptions to this rule as follows:

(a) Almost all jurisdictions now have special provisions for the treatment of certain conditions without the consent of the minor's parents. These conditions usually include drug abuse and venereal disease (contraception, abortion, and mental illness are sometimes included, and at other times, specifically excluded). Physicians should be aware of the provisions of the law in the jurisdiction in which they practice.

(b) The emancipated minor is a young person who lives independently of parents, physically, financially, or otherwise. Married minors, those in the armed forces, or those living away at college are considered emancipated. They may request treatment and be treated without parental consent.

(c) The legal concept of "mature minor" is increasingly invoked. A mature minor is one who is below statutory age and who is still dependent upon parents but who appears to make reasoned judgments. These young persons pose something of a quandary to the physician from whom they seek care. On the one hand, they appear able to decide for themselves; on the other hand, their parents remain legally responsible for them. Legal authorities conclude that the physician may respond to their requests under the following conditions: (1) The patient is at the age of discretion (15 years or older) and appears able to understand the procedure and its risks sufficiently to be able to give a genuinely informed consent; (2) the medical measures are taken for the patient's own benefit (i.e., not as a transplant donor or research subject); (3) the measures can be justified as necessary by medical opinion; and (4) there is some good reason, including simple refusal by the minor to request it, why parental consent cannot be obtained.

A physician may treat a minor without parental consent if the minor is emancipated or if there is statutory authorization for certain sorts of treatment. When the minor does not fit either category but is capable of understanding and consent, the physician may treat under the conditions mentioned previously. Physicians who honor the informed requests of mature minors for indicated treatment are at theoretical risk of parental challenge. However, legal opinion considers the risk to be minimal. In the case of the mature minor, however, the physician should inquire, if possible, about the reasons for the young person's unwillingness to communicate with parents. Steps should be taken, when the minor is willing, to attempt reconciliation or to solve the problem in a mutually satisfactory manner. Confidentiality should be maintained. Physicians should note that confidentiality is often unintentionally breached by billing procedures.

A request for irreversible sterilization from a mature minor poses special problems. Statutory and regulatory prohibitions against sterilization of minors are present in certain federal programs and in many states. A physician faces the possibility of a suit by parents and by the minor at a later date. One should assume that even a mature minor cannot comprehend the implications of this procedure. A physician confronted with this request should certainly explore the reasons behind the request and offer less radical alternatives.

Committee on Medical Liability, American Academy of Pediatrics. Elk Grove, IL, 1995.

2.7.5 P Parental Decisions Based on Religious or Cultural Beliefs

Parents are granted wide discretion about the values they believe their children's lives should embody. The constitutional protection of religious liberty safeguards this discretion particularly strongly. Yet, as a matter of course, state law and local courts have commonly intervened to prevent parents from exposing children to serious risk of life and health on the basis of religious beliefs. Nevertheless, the child abuse laws of many states specifically declare that a child is not to be deemed abused merely because he or she is being treated for illness by spiritual means, according to the tenets of a particular religion. Although often innocuous, these provisions sometimes put the life or health of a child in peril.

Case I. An 11-year-old girl is brought to an emergency department (ED) from an automobile accident. She is unconscious, with shallow, gasping respirations and circumoral cyanosis. Severe contusions are noted across the chest, the left side of which moves paradoxically on inspiration. She is hypotensive and tachycardic. An intravenous infusion of Ringer's lactate is started. After intubation and stabilization of BP, a chest film confirms flail chest and possible intrathoracic hemorrhage. Insertion of a chest tube produces frank blood. As the child is being wheeled toward the operating room, the parents, who had arrived minutes before, step in front of the gurney and declare that they are Jehovah's Witnesses and refuse permission for blood transfusion.

Case II. In 2.5.1 P, we saw Karen, a 13-year-old girl, refusing medical attention for suspected meningitis and supported by her parents in this refusal on the grounds of Christian Science beliefs. We recommended that her parents' decision be challenged and legal steps be taken, if necessary.

Case III. Also in Section 2.5.1 P, James, a 14-year-old boy with acute lymphocytic leukemia, refuses blood transfusions and is supported by his parents, who are Jehovah's Witnesses. We recommended that his refusal be respected.

Case IV. A 5-year-old child is brought to the emergency department (ED) by her parents, who are Hmong immigrants from Vietnam. The parents speak little English. The child has a high fever and fluid in the lungs. The ED resident notes that there are small circular burns on the child's chest and abdomen. She suspects child abuse.

COMMENT. Freedom of religion is highly valued and is protected by the Constitution of the United States. However, it is the freedom of the believer, capable of free and informed adherence to a faith, that is valued, not the effects of that belief on others, who do not or cannot accept it as their own. In the words of a Supreme Court decision about the authority of a Jehovah's Witness parent, "Parents may be free to become martyrs themselves, but it does not follow that they are free . . . to make martyrs of their children"(*Prince v Massachusetts*, 1944).

Even so, parents are given some latitude in determining appropriate treatments for their children. In a recent case, the Delaware Supreme Court permitted the Christian Scientist parents of a 3-year-old child suffering from Burkitt's lymphoma to refuse chemotherapy that had a 40%

chance of success. The court reasoned that the probability of success, when weighed against the parents' interests in directing the child's care and the possible harmful effects of the chemotherapy, was too low to justify forcing the child to undergo the medical treatment (*Newmark v Williams*, Delaware, 1991).

Neither of the two religious denominations mentioned previously considers that their children's souls will be damned by receiving medical treatment, nor is there any evidence that they consider their children tainted or excluded from their community. Even in states with religious exemptions, physicians and hospitals should be prepared to bring before the Child Protective Agency and to the courts any case involving "medical interventions of clear efficacy that can prevent, ameliorate, or cure serious disease, incapacity, or loss of life and interventions that will clearly result in prevention of future handicaps or disability for the child."

American Academy of Pediatrics Committee on Bioethics. Religious objections to medical care. *Pediatrics* 1997;99:279.

RECOMMENDATION. Blood transfusions should be initiated immediately in Case I. Court authority should be obtained only if delay will not jeopardize the child; otherwise, authority can be assumed on the basis of innumerable legal precedents allowing treatment in these conditions. In Case II, treatment should be started and authority sought to validate such a decision. Every effort should be made to placate the parents and maintain good relations, but the child's well-being, not the parents', is the issue. Case III, however, is different in an important way: The boy is old enough to understand and to have some personal commitments and the prognosis is poor, even with treatment. Transfusion will not cure, only palliate. It is ethical to omit transfusion in this case. In Case IV, the resident encounters a cultural practice common among the Hmong people. They place heated coins on the skin of a fevered patient, believing that the heat from the coins will draw out heat from the patient. The burns are small and superficial. Although parents might be dissuaded by education about this practice, it is not necessary to report abuse.

2.8 THE LIMITS OF PATIENT PREFERENCES

The preferences of patients have significant moral authority and must be considered in every treatment decision. Even the preferences of decisionally incapacitated patients are relevant to the decisions of those who must act in their behalf. However, the authority of patients' preferences is not unlimited. The ethical obligations of physicians are defined not only by the wishes of their patient but also by the goals of medicine.

Physicians have no obligation to perform actions beyond or contradictory to the goals of medicine, even when requested to do so by patients. Thus, patients have no right to demand that physicians provide medical care that is contraindicated, such as unnecessary surgery, or treatments that are unorthodox, such as eccentric drug regimens. Patients may not demand that physicians do anything illegal or unethical. For example, physicians must not provide certification of a disability that the patient does not have or fail to report communicable diseases at the patient's request. Finally, physicians may refuse to accede to a patient's wishes when deliberation convinces them that an ethical principle, other than respect for autonomy, takes priority in this situation, as we have shown in Chapter 1, with regard to beneficence and nonmaleficence, and as we will show in Chapter 4, with regard to fairness.

Traditionally, medical ethics has required physicians to abstain from moral judgments about their patients in regard to medical care. Two examples: (1) An ED physician is expected to provide competent care to both the wounded assailant of an elderly person and to the assaulted party; and (2) a physician should treat, without censure, venereal disease contracted in what the physician considers an immoral liaison. However, despite this professional neutrality, physicians and nurses have their own personal moral values. On occasion, they may be asked not merely to tolerate what they consider immorality but to participate in effecting an immoral action desired by the patient. Two examples: (1) A male patient requests a physician who considers transsexualism morally wrong, to prescribe female estrogens to promote secondary female characteristics; and (2) a Catholic nurse is asked to participate in an abortion. Usually, if there are laws pertaining to these subjects, explicit exemptions are noted for conscientious objection. Also, physicians may conscientiously judge that a particular law is unethical. For example, a physician treating AIDS patients is convinced that smoking marijuana relieves the pain and nausea of advanced illness, but state law prohibits prescription of "medical marijuana."

Physicians and nurses may refuse to cooperate in actions they judge immoral on grounds of conscience. It is important, in forming one's conscience, to separate the moral values to which one is committed from personal distaste or prejudice. For example, a physician refuses to undertake the care of a Jehovah's Witness with a hemorrhagic diathesis "on moral grounds," although, in fact, the physician does not like to feel impotent or run the risk of "losing a patient." Institutions and programs should establish policy about conscientious objection and make the policy clear to those who work in that institution or program. It is an accepted ethical principle that conscientious objection requires the objector to accept the consequences of violation of the law.

2.9 FAILURE TO COOPERATE WITH MEDICAL RECOMMENDATIONS

Physicians have the responsibility to recommend to patients a course of treatment or other behavior that would, in the physician's best judgment, help the patient. Patients have the right to be informed of the benefits and risks associated with these recommendations and to accept them or refuse them. These rights and responsibilities are in principle quite clear. However, patients may accept the recommendations of physicians and fail to act on them, yet continue to seek the care of the physician. This problem is known as "noncompliance" (a term that many dislike because of its paternalistic overtones). We prefer to use the expression "failure to cooperate with medical recommendations." The problem posed to physicians is how to perform their ethical responsibilities to patients who ask for help but for some reason do not, or cannot, avail themselves of what therapy is offered.

Case. Mr. Cope, a 42-year-old man with insulin-dependent diabetes, was first diagnosed at the age of 18 years. He complied with an insulin and dietary regimen faithfully. He nevertheless experienced frequent episodes of ketoacidosis and hypoglycemia, which necessitated repeated hospitalizations and emergency department care. For the past few years, his diabetes has been better controlled, and he required hospitalization only once for ketoacidosis associated with acute pyelonephritis. He has been actively involved in his diabetic program. He has been scrupulous about eating habits and has maintained an ideal body weight. He is knowledgeable about the use of insulin and currently takes 30 units of neutral protein Hagedorn insulin (NPH) and 10 units regular insulin each morning, and 15 units NPH in the evening. On this program, his urine fractionals are negative, his fasting blood sugars are less than 100 mg/dL, and his 2-hour postprandial sugars are usually less than 140 mg/dL. Twenty-one years after the onset of diabetes, he appears to have no functional impairment from his disease. Funduscopic examination reveals some neovascularization, which was treated with laser therapy, and urinalysis shows persistent proteinuria (less than 1 g/d). He has no neurologic or gastrointestinal symptoms.

After a stormy divorce and loss of an executive position, the patient has changed in several ways. In the 3 years after his divorce, he has gained 60 pounds and has become negligent about his insulin medication. He has also started to abuse alcohol excessively and had a serious automobile accident while driving under the influence. During these years, he has required frequent admissions to the hospital for diabetic complications, including (1) ketoacidosis, (2) traumatic and poorly healing foot ulcers, and (3) alcohol-related problems. While in the hospital, his diabetes is easier to manage but even in the hospital, he is frequently found in the cafeteria eating excessively. On two admissions, blood alcohol levels in excess of 200 mg/dL were detected. Soon after discharge from the hospital, his diabetic control lapses.

His physician is frustrated. He blames the recurring medical problems on the patient's unwillingness to participate actively in his own care. The physician tells him he could easily control his diabetic problem by merely resuming the same health habits he had pursued for so many years, that is, by losing weight, by taking his insulin regularly, and by drinking alcohol in moderation. The patient asserts that he will change his life style, but on discharge from the hospital, he relapses almost immediately. The physician urges him to seek psychiatric consultation. He agrees. The psychiatrist suggests a behavior modification program, which proves unsuccessful. Finally, aversion therapy is suggested. He refuses to participate in this program.

Mr. Cope continues to require hospitalization lasting 7 to 10 days every month or two. After 10 years of working closely with this patient, the physician considers withdrawing from the therapeutic relationship, because he senses he is no longer able to help the patient. "Why keep this up?" he says to the patient. "It's useless. Whatever I do, you undo." The patient resists this suggestion. He complains the physician is punishing him for drinking by abandoning him. Is persistent failure to comply with medical advice relevant to an ethical decision to withdraw from a case?

COMMENT. The following comments are relevant to this question:

(a) Patients such as Mr. Cope are very frustrating to those who attempt to care for them. Occasionally, the physician will accuse the patient (in words or in attitude) of being irresponsible. The patient engages constantly and apparently willfully in behavior that poses a serious risk to health and even to life. Such patients place great strain on the doctor-patient relationship; often the accommodation between doctor and patient founders because of the strain.

(b) The accusation of irresponsibility can be an example of the ethical fallacy of "blaming the victim"; the actual fault may lie with a more powerful party who finds a way to place the blame for his own failure on the ones who suffer its effects. The apparent irresponsibility of patients may be an impression created by the failure of a physician to educate, support, and convey a personal concern and interest in the patient. It may be more than an impression: Persons may be rendered incapable of caring responsibly for themselves by the way their physician deals with them. An excessive paternalism may stifle responsibility, while the physician's lack of personal concern may encourage tendencies to neglect medical advice. Although Mr. Cope's physician did not have these faults and had made solicitous efforts to support Mr. Cope, this problem may lie behind many cases of a patient's failure to cooperate.

RECOMMENDATIONS. (a) It is important to determine whether and to what extent the patient is acting voluntarily or involuntarily. Much uncooperative behavior is voluntary in the sense that the patient demonstrates no signs of pathologic behavior. Patients either choose to ignore the regimen in favor of other behaviors they value more than health (a goal that, in an asymptomatic disease, may not seem very urgent or immediate) or fail to cooperate because of such factors as irregular routine, complicated regimen, habitual forgetfulness, or poor explanation by the physician. Some noncompliance arises from profound emotional disturbance and ambivalence.

(b) If the physician judges that noncooperation is a result of the patient's persistence in voluntary health risks, reasonable efforts at rational persuasion should be undertaken. If these fail, it is ethically permissible for the physician to adjust therapeutic goals and do the best in the circumstance; it is also ethically permissible to withdraw from the case, after advising the patient how to obtain care from other sources.

(c) If contextual features, such as inability to pay for medicines, inadequate housing, and so forth, are the reasons for noncooperation, help should be provided to improve these circumstances.

(d) If noncooperation is the result of a psychologic disorder, the physician has a strong ethical obligation to remain with the patient, adjusting treatment plans to the undesirable situation. Professional assistance in treating the disorder should be sought. The physician will experience great frustration, but the frustration is not, in itself, sufficient to justify leaving the patient.

2.9.1 The Problem Patient: Noncritical

Failure to cooperate with medical recommendations occurs in situations where the results, although harmful to the health of the patient, are not critical.

Case. Mr. Cope was admitted for inpatient treatment of obesity with a protein-sparing modified fasting regimen. He was found repeatedly in the cafeteria cheating on the diet. His physician made reasonable efforts to persuade him to change his behavior.

RECOMMENDATION. It would be ethically permissible for the physician to abandon therapeutic goals and to discharge the patient from the hospital. These goals are unachievable because of the patient's failure to participate in the treatment program.

2.9.2 The Problem Patient: Critically Ill

Is it ever justifiable to discharge a "problem patient" who has a critical illness requiring in-hospital treatment? Just as we believe that noncritically ill patients can be discharged if they repeatedly frustrate physicians' efforts to provide needed medical assistance, we also believe that noncooperation that directly counters the physician's effort can justify discharging a patient who is critically ill and in need of care. The situation, however, is more serious and requires added considerations before a decisive conclusion can be reached.

Case. R.A., an intravenous drug addict, is admitted for the third time in 3 years with a diagnosis of infective endocarditis. Three years before, he required mitral valve replacement for *Pseudomonas* endocarditis, and 1 year ago, he required replacement of the prosthetic valve after he developed *Staphylococcus aureus* endocarditis. He now is admitted again with *S aureus* endocarditis of the prosthetic valve.

After 1 week of antibiotic therapy, he continues to have positive blood cultures. He consents to open heart surgery to replace again the infected prosthetic mitral valve. For 10 days postoperatively (4 days in the ICU) he is cooperative with his management and antibiotic treatment. On this treatment he becomes afebrile, and blood cultures are negative.

He then begins to behave erratically. He leaves his room and stays away for hours, often missing his medications. On several occasions, a urine screening test demonstrates the presence of opiates and quinine, suggesting that he is using illicit narcotics even while being treated for infective endocarditis. On two separate occasions he punches nurses who scold him for being away from his room. On the eleventh postoperative day, he is discovered by hospital security guards in his bathroom selling injectable narcotics to another patient. His roommate in the hospital had observed these dealings for several days, but the patient threatened to kill the roommate if he told anyone about these transactions. When all this information becomes known to the patient's physician, the patient is asked to leave the hospital immediately. Despite the fact that the patient's infective endocarditis has not been treated optimally, he was discharged from the hospital against his will.

COMMENT. Considerations leading to an ethical justification of this decision are as follows:

(a) The patient's use of intravenous street drugs at the same time that his physicians were attempting to eradicate his infective endocarditis indicated that the likelihood of medical success in this case, both short-term and long-term, was not great. Physicians are not obliged to treat people who persist in actions that run directly counter to the goals of such treatment.

(b) The patient wanted to be treated and, at the same time, continued his abusive and illegal behavior. The physicians are obliged to determine that the patient has the mental capacity to make such choices and that he was not suffering from a metabolic encephalopathy (see Section 2.2). On the other hand, the physicians are not obliged to deal with the patient's long-standing sociopathic behavior pattern.

(c) This patient's physicians (who were hospital-based) had obligations both to this patient and to their other hospitalized patients. This patient's behavior of selling narcotics to other inpatients and of terrorizing his roommate compromised the care other patients of the same physician were receiving. This patient, then, posed a direct and serious threat to other identifiable persons. He is also engaged in criminal behavior.

RECOMMENDATION. Mr. R.A. is not only a difficult patient; he is also dangerous. The ethical obligation to protect others, both patients and staff, from his behavior overrides the obligation to provide him with medical care. Recourse to legal authorities is advisable. Providers should try to understand the complex causes of his behavior and motivations. They should avoid "blaming the victim." Serious efforts should be made to counsel, to negotiate, and to develop "contracts" that make clear to him the consequences of his behavior. Early and repeated warnings should be issued. One identified provider should be responsible for dealing with this patient. Yet, the protection of other persons and the observance of the law are predominant in this case.

2.9.3 The Problem Patient: Socially Unacceptable

Some patients with critical illnesses are difficult to care for because providers find them personally repugnant and judge them to be the cause of their own illness. Such persons are often destitute and considered "socially unacceptable."

Case. A 35-year-old chronic alcoholic with a long criminal record had an emergency portacaval shunt for variceal bleeding. He continued to drink alcohol. One year after his operation, he was admitted twice within 3 months with acute bleeding from esophageal varices.

COMMENT. There are two problems with this patient. First, there is the suspicion that he will appear again, in the near future, with the same problem. Second, his problem was caused by personal behavior that is socially unacceptable. The first problem presents the issues in Chapter 4 about allocation of scarce resources (Section 4.4); when the patient does become a repeater, the considerations mentioned there are relevant to a decision about his treatment. The second problem is discussed under quality of life (Section 3.0.5). It should be noted that some harmful personal habits are commonly considered more socially unacceptable than others. Substance abuse is strongly disapproved, whereas overeating, fast driving, not wearing seatbelts, or engaging in dangerous sports is tolerated or even praised. Many conditions requiring expensive medical treatment are caused by behaviors that are socially accepted. Thus, singling out socially disapproved behaviors as less deserving of treatment reflects social prejudices rather than logic.

RECOMMENDATION. This patient should be managed with aggressive medical and surgical means in an effort to control his hemorrhage and to reverse his blood loss. A patient's past behavior is not sufficient reason to warrant physicians' withdrawal from the treatment of serious illness. In most cases, the patient's past history should be ignored except insofar as it is medically relevant. Refusal to treat a patient can be ethically justified in view of a person's behavior in the present circumstances only when that behavior makes achievement of medical goals impossible.

2.9.4 Signing Out against Medical Advice

Mr. R.A., the patient described in Section 2.9.2, might leave the hospital before physicians judge his treatment adequate. When patients choose to discharge themselves in this manner, most hospitals request them to sign a statement confirming that they are leaving against medical advice (AMA). The patients, however, cannot be forced to sign the statements; they have the right to leave at will. The document merely provides legal evidence that the patient's departure was voluntary and that the patient was warned by the physician about the risks of leaving. This warning, performed as patiently and carefully as possible, is the ethical duty of the physician.

2.9.5 Withdrawing from the Case and Abandonment

At times, such as the case of Mr. Cope (Section 2.9), the physician may serve the patient best by deciding to dissolve the physician-patient relationship and by helping the patient to find another physician. The physician's principal goal is to help patients in the care of their health. If, for whatever reasons, this proves impossible, the physician may best demonstrate ethical responsibility by withdrawing from the case and finding another physician who might be more successful with the patient in these particular circumstances.

Physicians who terminate the relationship with a patient sometimes wonder whether they can be charged with "abandonment." A legal charge of abandonment can be brought when the physician, without giving timely notice, ceases to provide care for a patient who is still in need of medical attention or when the physician is dilatory and careless (e.g., failure to visit the patient in the hospital or failure to judge the patient's condition serious enough to warrant attention). A charge of abandonment can usually be countered by showing that the patient did receive warning in sufficient time to arrange for medical care. The physician is not legally obliged to arrange for further care from another physician, although there is a legal obligation to provide full medical records to the new attending physician. If the physician does intend to maintain the relationship with the patient but will be unavailable for a time, there is a legal obligation to arrange for coverage by another physician. Failure to do so can be construed as abandonment.

Thus, a physician may withdraw from the care of a patient without legal risk. Still, a decision to do so should meet ethical as well as legal standards. Physicians inherit an ethical tradition that requires them to undertake difficult tasks and even risks for the care of persons in need of medical attention. Inconvenience, provocation, or dislike are not sufficient reasons to exempt a physician from that duty. That obligation is, of course, limited by several conditions. If the patient absorbs excessive time and energy, drawing the physician away from other patients, if the patient is acting in ways to frustrate the attainable medical goals, or if the patient is endangering others by overt action, the ethical obligation to continue to care would be diminished. These conditions appear to be verified in the case of Mr. R.A.

2.10 ALTERNATIVE MEDICINE

Many persons seek care from providers who are not trained in conventional scientific medicine. These providers apply physical, psychologic, and herbal remedies that are not commonly recognized as scientific or proven effective by clinical trials. The most common of these providers are naturopaths, homeopaths, chiropractors, and acupuncturists. States license these practitioners, and in several states, homeopathic and naturopathic doctors are licensed as medical practitioners. Methods include spiritual healing, physical manipulation, special diets, imaging, relaxation techniques, massage, and vitamin therapy. These methods are described as "alternative" or "complementary" medicine. Often patients who are under the care of regular practitioners are also seeking care from these alternative practitioners. What then is the obligation of the physician toward such patients?

Adams KE, Cohen MH, Eisenberg D, Jonsen AR. Ethical considerations of complementary and alternative medical therapies in conventional medical settings. *Ann Intern Med* 2002;137:660–664.

Case. A 64-year-old man has been under the care of a family physician for increasingly severe osteoarthritis. On one visit, he complains of dizzy spells. A workup reveals no specific cause for his dizziness. In discussing his arthritis, he tells his doctor that he gets some relief from mushroom tea. The physician has seen reports of illness caused by "kombucha tea," which, although called "mushroom tea," is actually a colony of bacteria and yeast fermented in sweetened tea. The physician questions the patient, and the patient reluctantly admits that he has been seeing a "natural healer" who sold him the concoction.

McNaughton C, Eidsness LM. Ethics of alternative therapies. *S D J Med* 1995;48:209–211.

COMMENT. The large number of persons who visit alternative practitioners (estimated to be about one of every three adult Americans, making some 425 million visits yearly—more than are made to regular primary care practitioners) commonly do so in conjunction with care from regular practitioners, using unconventional therapies as adjuncts rather than replacements of conventional therapy. The majority of these patients do not inform their regular physician about their use of alternative treatment. Preferences for alternative treatments are often motivated because they are less arduous and less costly than conventional treatments, or because patients are frustrated with the failure of conventional treatment to assuage problems such as chronic back pain, headache, insomnia, anxiety, and depression. Most conventional practitioners know little about alternative medicine, and many commonly disdain it and disparage its claims.

RECOMMENDATION. (a) Conventional physicians should encourage their patients to reveal their use of alternative medications; disparaging remarks inhibit patients from speaking about what they fear will lead to anger or ridicule on the physician's part.

(b) Conventional physicians should try to attain a better understanding of the healing systems to which patients have frequent recourse and to appreciate their beneficial features. The risks of some commonly used substances, such as St. Johns Wort, are known and should be familiar to physicians. Efforts are being made to submit many of these therapies to scientific evaluation in controlled trials.

(c) When patients are using alternative therapies for serious conditions to the neglect of demonstrated efficacious therapies, or when they are using therapies that have toxic effects, physicians should carefully explain the consequences of such a course. A clumsy or uninformed approach may confirm patients in the use of inadvisable therapy rather than convert them to the physician's recommended ones.

(d) In serious conditions, where the use of alternative medicine may impede cure or be dangerous, the physician should ask the patient's permission to contact the alternative provider, explain the situation, and negotiate a program that will be acceptable to the patient and conformable to the ethics of the providers.

(e) Hospitals should develop policies that acknowledge the prevalence of alternative therapies and establish guidelines for acceptable collaboration between regular physicians and providers of alternative treatments.

Chapter 3

3.0
Quality of Life

Quality of life is the third topic that must be reviewed to analyze a problem in clinical ethics. After reviewing medical indications and patient preferences, the patient's quality of life before the current illness and expected quality of life with or without treatment should be described. This chapter is devoted to explaining the difficult concept of quality of life, analyzing its implications for clinical decisions, and suggesting certain distinctions and cautions that should be observed in discussing the concept in the context of clinical care.

The most fundamental goal of medical care is the improvement of the quality of life for all those who need and seek care. All of the more particular goals stated in Section 1.0.2, such as relief of pain and improvement of function, are aspects of this one fundamental objective. Patients seek medical attention because they are distressed by symptoms, worried by doubts about their health, or disabled by accidents and disease. The physician responds by examining, evaluating, diagnosing, treating, curing, comforting, and educating. These activities aim at improvement of the quality of the patient's life.

In many clinical situations, that improvement can be effected easily and rapidly. For example, Mr. Cure's headache, stiff neck, and malaise are symptoms of meningitis and can be relieved by administering an antibiotic that will eliminate the infection causing them. The quality of his life, impaired by the infection, is rapidly restored to normal. In other situations, the quality of the patient's life is seriously disrupted by a disease for which no cure is available; the patient will become progressively disabled. Medical intervention aims at reduction of discomfort and maintenance of normal functions to the extent possible. For example, the quality of life for Mrs. Care, who has multiple sclerosis, is generally diminished but made "tolerable" by various medical, nursing, and rehabilitative interventions. In other situations, a patient's disease may be treated by an intervention that may cure the disease or retard its progress but, at the same time, reduce the quality of the patient's life. For example, Mr. Cope, a patient with brittle diabetes, will have to endure a strict dietary and insulin regimen and Ms. Comfort will have to undergo a mastectomy and multiple courses of chemotherapy and radiotherapy in the attempt to conquer her cancer.

The evaluation of quality of life is always relevant to appropriate medical care. Physicians and patients must determine what level of quality is desirable, how it is to be attained, and what risks and disadvantages are associated with the desired level. Unlike the risks and benefits considered in medical interventions, which are relatively immediate, quality-of-life considerations focus on the long-term consequences of accepting or refusing a recommendation for medical intervention. These considerations should be a part of all serious discussions of medical choices. However, they raise ethical questions in several ways: (1) when there is a notable divergence between quality of life as assessed by physicians and by patients, (2) when patients are unable to express their evaluation of the quality of life they wish to have, (3) when the enhancement of normal qualities is sought as a goal of medicine, and (4) when quality of life is used as an objective standard for rationing of care. The first three issues are discussed in this chapter; the fourth is discussed in Chapter 4.

Beauchamp TL, Childress JF. The centrality of quality of life judgments. In: *Principles of Biomedical Ethics.* 5th ed. New York: Oxford University Press; 2001:136–139.

Beauchamp TL, Childress JF. The value and quality of life. In: *Principles of Biomedical Ethics.* 5th ed. New York: Oxford University Press; 2001:206–212.

3.0.1 Meaning of Quality of Life

Despite the importance of quality of life in clinical medicine, the phrase is not easy to define. The phrase expresses a value judgment: The experience of living, as a whole or in some aspect, is judged to be "good" or "bad," "better," or "worse." In recent years, efforts have been made to develop measures of quality of life that can be used to evaluate outcomes of clinical interventions. Such measures list a variety of physical functions, such as mobility, performance of activities of daily living, absence or presence of pain, social interaction, and mental acuity. Scales are devised to rate the range of performance and satisfaction with these aspects of living. These various measures attempt to provide an objective description of what is inevitably a highly subjective and personal evaluation. Also, many surveys inquiring about personal appraisal of quality of life and that of others have been made. Even when measures are based on empirical surveys of what persons consider valuable, individuals may depart, often in striking ways, from the general view. Empirical studies of this subject are difficult to design and are limited in application.

Quality-of-life judgments, then, are not based on a single dimension, nor are they entirely subjective or objective. They must consider personal and social function and performance, symptoms, prognosis, and the subjective values that patients ascribe to quality of life. Several important questions must be addressed: (1) Who is making the evaluation—the person living the life or an observer? (2) What criteria are being used for evaluation? And finally, the crucial ethical question: (3) What types of clinical decisions, if any, are justified by reference to quality-of-life judgments? Occasionally, a distinction is made between sanctity of life and quality of life. Those who make this distinction may wish to claim that human life is so valuable that it must be preserved at all costs, under any conditions, and for as long as possible. This view has deep roots in some religious traditions. It also has a secular counterpart, called "vitalism," that is sometimes encountered in medicine: Organic life must be preserved even when all other human functions are lost. It is our belief that the profound respect for human life expressed in the phrase "sanctity of life" is compatible with the view that seriously diminished quality of life may justify refraining from medical treatments that pro-long life.

3.0.2 Distinctions

It is important to distinguish between two uses of the phrase "quality of life." Failure to do so can cause confusion in clinical discussions.

(a) One interpretation of the phrase is the personal satisfaction expressed or experienced by individuals in their physical, mental, and social situation. We call this "personal evaluation." This personal evaluation of an individual's own quality of life is an essential component of patient preferences, as we have explained in Chapter 2. In this sense, ethical questions about quality of life are generally equivalent to the ethics of personal autonomy.

EXAMPLE I. A 27-year-old gymnastics instructor who is paralyzed because of a cervical spinal cord lesion may say, "My life isn't as bad as it looks: I've come to terms with my loss and discovered the powers of the mind."

EXAMPLE II. A 68-year-old artist who is a diabetic now faces blindness and multiple amputations. She says, "I wonder if I can endure a life of such poor quality?"

(b) Another interpretation of the phrase is the evaluation by an on-looker of another's experiences of personal life. We call this "observer evaluation." Quality of life, understood in this sense, produces the many ethical problems that are explored in this chapter.

EXAMPLE III. A parent says of a 29-year-old retarded son with an IQ score of 40, "He used to seem so happy, but now he's become so restless and difficult—what kind of quality of life does he have?"

EXAMPLE IV. An 83-year-old woman with advanced senile dementia, who is bedridden and tube-fed, is described by the nurses as "having poor quality of life."

COMMENT. Reference to quality of life in a clinical discussion is natural and necessary, but because the phrase can be used in so many ways, its use can cause confusion. Several distinctions must be made as follows:

(a) The judgment of poor quality of life may be made by the one who lives the life (personal evaluation) or by an observer (observer evaluation). It often happens that lives that observers consider of poor quality are lived quite satisfactorily by the one living that life. Human beings are amazingly adaptive. They can make the best of the options available. For example, the quadriplegic gymnastics instructor may be a person of extraordinary motivation, the blind artist may enjoy a vivid imagination, and the developmentally disabled person may enjoy simple pleasures. Thus, if patients can evaluate and express their own quality of life, other parties should not presume to judge but should seek the patients' opinions. Similarly, when the person's own evaluation is not or cannot be known to others, those others should be extremely cautious in applying their own values.

(b) Poor quality of life might mean, in general, that the sufferer's experiences fall below some standard that the speaker considers desirable. But in each case, the experience in question is different; it may be pain, loss of mobility, presence of multiple debilitating health problems, loss of mental capacity and of the enjoyment of human interaction, loss of joy in life, and so on. Poor quality of life, then, refers to many quite different circumstances.

(c) Evaluation of the quality of life, like life itself, changes with time. The artist's concern may be the result of a temporary depression that will resolve as she discovers her future possibilities; the gymnastics instructor may later become deeply depressed. Thus, providers of care must be careful not to make momentous decisions on the basis of possibly transitory conditions.

(d) The evaluation may reflect bias and prejudice. When sufferers from mental retardation are said to have "poor quality of life," this may reflect our cultural bias in favor of intelligence and productivity. Prejudice may incline some people to judge that persons of a certain ethnic origin, social status, or sexual preference cannot possibly have "good quality" of life.

(e) The evaluation may reflect socioeconomic conditions rather than the experienced life of the patient, for example, the lack of home care, of rehabilitation, or of special education. These obstacles, while very real, can often be overcome by planning and effort on the part of providers.

EXAMPLE. Dax Cowart, described in the Introduction, believed at first that his disabilities caused by the explosion—blindness, disfigurement, crippling—would make his life intolerable and not worth living. He wanted to refuse treatment and be allowed to die. His personal assessment of his quality of life was that it was too poor to go on living. Later, Dax revised his earlier assessment as he gradually learned to appreciate mental activities, to enjoy the pleasures of music, and to cope with his frustrations. He became a lecturer about his own story and an advocate for the rights of patients and the disabled. He graduated from law school, passed the bar, and now practices law. He continues to deal daily with frustrations of his disabilities, but he has achieved a quality of life that he could not previously have imagined. Many persons, on viewing the videotape *Please Let Me Die,* where Dax is shown at a time of extreme distress and deficits, judge his life to be of such poor quality that it could not be worth living. He would have agreed at that time, but now he views his life differently (although he still believes that he should not have been deprived of the right to end his life). In addition to Dax's personal assessment, those who provided care for him—physicians, surgeons, and nurses—offered observer assessments that were more optimistic than Dax's. They had seen patients equally badly burned recover to an acceptable quality of life and tended to impose this experience on Dax. This example reminds us of the need for caution in applying quality-of-life judgments in clinical decisions.

Confronting death: Who chooses? Who decides? A dialogue between Dax Cowart and Robert Burt. *Hastings Cent Rep* 1998;28(1):14–28.

3.0.3 Best Interest Standard and Quality of Life

At Section 2.7.2, we noted that when authorized persons, such as next-of-kin, guardians, or parties holding durable powers of attorney, make decisions for the patients, they are required to follow previously known wishes of the patients or, if their wishes are not known, to act in their best interests. The concept of **best interest**, drawn from legal parlance, is often difficult to apply to health care situations. In general, it refers to the quality of life that a "reasonable person" would choose were he or she able to do so. "Reasonable person" is a useful fiction, devised to express what we might expect the priorities of most human beings to be in a typical situation. This is quite vague. Two clarifications might be helpful. First, what counts as an interest should be designated, as much as possible, from the viewpoint of the one for whom the judgment is being made. The interests common to competent, intelligent persons may not even occur to persons who suffer significant limitations of these faculties. Still, they have interests in the pursuit and securing of certain values suited to their limitations. The proxy decision makers should attempt to view the world of such persons through their eyes. Second, when evidence of just how these persons would view the world is absent, the interests at stake should be judged by reference to critically assessed, societally shared values. Critical assessment consists in scrutinizing societally shared values for misinformation, prejudice, discrimination, and stereotyping.

3.0.4 Divergent Evaluations of Quality of Life

Because evaluation of quality of life is so subjective, different observers will rate certain forms of living quite differently. This can introduce bias and even discrimination into judgments and may affect clinical care adversely. Four major problems of this sort appear in clinical ethics: (1) lack of understanding about the patient's own values, (2) divergence between physicians' assessment of patients' quality of life and the assessments made by patients themselves, (3) bias and discrimination that negatively affect the physician's dedication to the patient's welfare, and (4) the introduction of social worth criteria into quality-of-life judgments.

Studies have shown that physicians consistently rate the quality of life of their patients lower than do the patients themselves. In one study, physicians and patients were asked independently to evaluate living with certain chronic conditions, such as arthritis, ischemic heart disease, chronic pulmonary disease, and cancer. Physicians judged life with these conditions to be less tolerable than did the patients who suffered from them. Physicians based their assessments primarily on disease conditions, whereas patients also took into account nonmedical factors, such as interpersonal relationships, finances, and social conditions. Also, studies have shown that physicians' quality-of-life assessments do influence important clinical decisions such as those about resuscitation.

EXAMPLE. A 62-year-old man with metastatic colon cancer has been doing relatively well until he is diagnosed with uremia secondary to obstructive nephropathy. He is encephalopathic. The physician believes that uremia is a quiet way to die, while advancing metastatic disease would be very distressing. He recommends that the obstruction not be relieved. The patient's wife insists on surgical treatment. The patient recovered and lived an additional 10 months with satisfactory quality of life until 2 weeks before his death.

COMMENT. This sort of divergence in evaluation can lead to serious misjudgments about the appropriateness of therapy. It is essential that physicians discuss the issue of quality of life with the patient and attempt to determine as explicitly as possible the values held by the patient. Physicians should become more adept in discussing these elusive matters with patients; the use of "values histories" may be helpful.

3.0.5 Bias and Discrimination

One of the important ethical achievements of medicine in the tradition of Western culture is the tenet that those in need should be cared for regardless of race, religion, or nationality. Individual physicians, however, may have beliefs and values that lead to biased and discriminatory judgments against certain persons or classes of persons. These judgments may affect clinical decisions. (a) Racial Bias. The history of American medicine is stained by discrimination against African-Americans and Native Americans. Today these biases may be less explicit but no less harmful. It is ethically important that they be identified and eliminated from clinical decisions.

Bioethics and race. *Hastings Cent Rep;* 2001;31:5.

(b) Bias against the Elderly and the Disabled. Studies have revealed that many physicians, particularly younger ones, are biased against elderly patients. They are reluctant to deal with them and sometimes make prejudicial judgments about them.

Case. A 92-year-old woman is brought unconscious to the emergency department (ED). On examination, she is unresponsive, dehydrated, and hypotensive. She is also found to have a urinary tract infection and pulmonary infiltrates, possibly caused by aspiration. The ED resident believes she has sepsis from a urinary tract source but wonders whether to start antibiotics and fluid resuscitation because of her reported age. The attending physician orders treatment. On recovery, the patient returns to her previous rather vigorous and alert quality of life, which had not been known to the treating physicians.

COMMENT. Treatment decisions should be based on medical need and presumed patient preference. Discrimination against persons on the basis of their chronological age is morally wrong. Even if a person's contribution to society is considered important, it is not, in itself, the criterion of a just and fair distribution of social benefits. Age is not an accurate indicator of the extent of contribution to society. Contributions may be made in many ways other than economic productivity, and present social goods are built on past contributions.

(c) Lifestyle Bias. Studies have revealed that physicians are no more free of bias against certain life styles than the general population. In particular, negative attitudes or discomfort at homosexual identity has been noted. One 1987 study showed that, in a sample of physicians, a significant number of physicians stigmatized patients identified as gay and showed less willingness to interact with them even in ordinary conversation. This bias can seriously affect the care of homosexual men with HIV infection and AIDS. Although a decade of experience may have mitigated this bias, some providers may still harbor these attitudes.

(d) Gender Bias. Gender bias exists, overtly or covertly, throughout our society. In health care, it has been demonstrated that male physicians discount women's health complaints and that research has been designed in ways that fail to appropriately evaluate treatments for women. Prejudices often discount the intelligence and autonomy of women.

Tong R. An introduction to feminist approaches to bioethics: Unity in diversity. *J Clin Ethics* 1996;7(1):13–19.

Tong R. Feminist approaches to bioethics. *J Clin Ethics* 1996;7(4):315–319.

(e) Social Worth. Judgments about quality of life should be directed primarily to the characteristics and experiences of individuals. However, it is easy to include in such judgments beliefs about how persons with a certain quality of life contribute, or fail to contribute, to the social community of which they are a part. This may be legitimate, or it may be extremely prejudicial and unfair.

RECOMMENDATION. In general, social worth criteria are not relevant to diagnosis and treatment of particular patients. Patients should not be afforded or refused treatment on the basis of social worth. It is not the physician's prerogative to make such judgments in the context of providing medical treatment: Criminals, addicts, and enemies should be treated in relation to their medical need, not their social worth. The impact of a patient's socioeconomic situation may be relevant, however, to prognosis and eligibility for special services, such as organ transplantation. Transplantation, for example, may require the ability and willingness to undergo rigorous follow-up. Occasionally, social worth may be relevant in certain triage situations. On these points, see Section 4.4.2.

3.0.6 The Disagreeable Patient

In Section 2.9, several patients were described who had characteristics that made it difficult to care for them. Mr. Cope was uncooperative, alcoholic, and unpleasant. Another patient was an abusive drug addict. A third was a habitual criminal. Health care providers may find such patients exasperating, disagreeable, and even repugnant. This reaction may distort clinical decisions about such patients and affect the quality of care provided to them. Providers should make strenuous efforts to overcome their negative attitudes toward such patients.

EXAMPLE. Mr. C.D. is an alcoholic who inhabits building excavations. He is extremely filthy, foul-mouthed, and, at times, violent and disruptive. He appears quite regularly at the hospital in need of various sorts of care for pneumonia, frostbite, delirium tremens, and so forth. One of the house officers, despite a reprimand from the chief resident, persists in calling him Gomer the Gopher. He is brought to the ED for the third time in a month with bleeding esophageal varices. The ED intern says, "High quality of life like Gomer's we can do without."

COMMENT. Mr. C.D.'s quality of life, while certainly poor with respect to the values of our culture, is not relevant to medical decisions. He does, however, impose certain burdens on his providers and on society that may be relevant to judgments about his care. This contextual factor is considered in Chapter 4.

3.0.7 Developmental Disability

Persons whose lives are limited as a result of developmental disability are often objects of discrimination. Given the range of possibilities for social intercourse, intellectual achievement, personal accomplishment, and productivity open to most human beings, the lives of these persons seem severely restricted. It might be said, then, that they live lives of diminished quality. When decisions about medical care are made for such persons, is such diminished quality of life a relevant consideration?

EXAMPLE. Mr. A.T. is a 67-year-old man who has been institutionalized for severe developmental disability since he was 1 year old. His mental age is estimated at less than the 3-year-old level, and his IQ score is 10. He develops acute myelogenous leukemia. His guardian says, "His life is of such poor quality. Why should we try to extend it?"

COMMENT. The above case recalls one in which an important legal decision was rendered. In that case, the Massachusetts Supreme Court approved a decision not to treat Joseph Saikewicz, a 67-year-old developmentally disabled man, with chemotherapy. The court attempted to distinguish between the quality of life of the developmentally disabled, which it did not consider relevant to the decision, and the quality of life that Joseph Saikewicz "was likely to experience" under treatment. Speaking of the continued state of pain and disorientation likely to result from chemotherapy, the courts said, "he would experience fear without the understanding from which other patients draw strength." This distinction suggests a point of ethical importance. Deciding to withhold medical treatment from an individual because that individual belongs to a class of persons whose lives are limited when judged by social norms for accomplishment and productivity is ethically dangerous. Such decisions look more to the burden these persons place on society than to the burden these persons themselves experience. The peril of seeing persons as class members for the purpose of medical treatment is a "slippery slope"; that is, it is starting a process in which classes of "undesirables" grow increasingly wider and take in more and more persons who are "burdens to themselves and others."

3.0 P Features of Quality-of-Life Judgments for Infants and Children

Two important differences distinguish these judgments from those in adult care. First, the adult often can express preferences about future states of life and health. Second, when an adult is incapable of expressing preferences, the history of that person's preferences and style of life often allows others to estimate how that person would value and adapt to future states. In pediatrics, the life whose quality is being assessed is almost entirely in the future, and no expression of preferences is available. Just as in adult care, pediatricians tend to assess quality of life as lower than either parents or the children with the condition.

Special Issue. Imperiled Newborns. *Hastings Cent Rep* 1987;17.

Special Issue. Neonatal Ethics. *J Clin Ethics* 2001;12(3).

Case I. Peter, a 12-year-old boy with Down's syndrome, has had a congenital heart lesion, known since birth. No surgical intervention was recommended until he was 12 years old. Peter's IQ tests at the higher end of the range common to Down's syndrome. He is now a Boy Scout, active in sports and an average performer in special school. His parents refuse permission for surgery that would effect normal longevity, saying that after they died, his quality of life would be intolerable.

Case II. A newborn infant is noted to have the stigmata of Down's syndrome, which is confirmed by chromosome studies. He also suffers from duodenal atresia, for which immediate surgery is indicated. His parents refuse permission, saying that the baby was better dead than living the life of a retarded person.

COMMENT. The perils of quality-of-life judgment are demonstrated in these cases. In Case I, the judgment is about a far future and does not reflect Peter's relative success in dealing with his limitation. The judgment of Peter's parents does not reflect significant facts about their son's life and, at the same time, has implications of great consequence and certain outcome for their son. Deprived of the recommended surgery, he will continue to live for some time and slowly develop the debilitating effects of severe cardiac insufficiency and pulmonary hypertension. In Case II, a general predisposition to devalue limited intelligence, achievement, productivity, and independence colors judgment. These social values, while highly valued in our culture, are not the only human values. They are not so important that their invocation should lead to death for those who can attain them in only limited degree.

RECOMMENDATION. Medical interventions that are generally effective in alleviating physical disability are ethically mandatory when the only supposed contraindication is developmental disabilities in the range characteristic of Down's syndrome. More complicated medical conditions, such as major cardiac deformity, may be genuine contraindications, but for the same reasons that they may contraindicate surgery for an otherwise normal infant.

3.0.1 P Best Interest Standard for Children

Children have no history of preferences on which to base a surrogate judgment. Thus, the first standard for surrogate decisions, substituted judgment, is not relevant; all surrogate judgments for minor children must adhere to the best interest standard (Section 3.0.3).

Case I. Monica, born at term, is noted at birth to have a large thoracolumbar myelomeningocele that is leaking cerebrospinal fluid. In addition to extreme kyphosis, Monica appears to be microcephalic. Computerized tomography of the head shows cerebral dysgenesis and ventriculomegaly, with a cortical mantle of less than 5 mm. Monica's parents, who understand the situation, request that no medical interventions be performed. They wish to take Monica home to die.

Case II. An 1100-g premature male infant, born at 32 weeks' gestational age, is now 2 days old and in the recovery phase of moderately severe hyaline membrane disease. A drop in hematocrit and a prolonged indirect hyperbilirubinemia suggest occult bleeding. A cranial ultrasound study confirms a grade III intraventricular hemorrhage. After being informed of the possible risks of mental retardation, the infant's parents request that the mechanical ventilation be stopped.

Case III. John is a 2-day-old infant who was started on a prostaglandin infusion when an echocardiogram confirmed that a hypoplastic left heart was the cause of his poor pulses. To control respiratory distress and reduce the work of breathing, John was intubated, ventilated, and sedated. The neonatologists are pleased with how John has stabilized in response to their management. They discuss the various options with John's parents. This intelligent young couple begin by saying they want John to have as normal a life as possible, but express their concern about putting him through suffering to achieve it.

COMMENT. In Case I, the prognosis includes severe deformity of the spine and lower limbs, incontinence of bowel and bladder, and the near certainty of profound mental retardation. Multiple surgical procedures will be required during early life for orthopedic problems, and there is high likelihood of frequent infection of bladder catheter and ventriculoperitoneal shunt. Monica will never be able to understand and communicate. The combination of extreme and painful disabilities and severe retardation constitutes a quality of life that can confidently be judged to be undesirable for, and undesired by, any human being. In Case II, there is significant probability of disability, although the extent is unpredictable. There may be some residual chronic lung deficiencies. The ethical difference between Cases I and II lies in the reliable predictability for Monica of a life of physical pain without even the solace of experiencing the compassion of others and of understanding one's own condition; for John, only an uncertain prediction of mental or physical limitation can be made. The judgment of quality of life in the first case invokes a condition that can confidently be evaluated as one that any human being would wish to avoid. The situation described in Case II affords no such confidence. The criteria for judging treatment to be in the child's best interest are more applicable to Case II than to Case I.

In Case III, there are only three options for John's care. Because a hypoplastic left heart is incompatible with life, the parents may choose to allow John to die. They may, however, choose a staged surgical repair of the heart, known as the Norwood procedure. Currently, some two-thirds of infants survive up to 5 years after three operations performed over the first 3 years of life. At the same time, many of these infants suffer from major developmental disabilities as complications of surgery or hospitalization. A final option is heart transplantation, but the long wait, because of the shortage of organs, makes this an unlikely option.

RECOMMENDATION. We propose that a decision to refrain from intervention that is designed to prolong life is ethically justified in Case I, but not in Case II. The federal Baby Doe rules state that life-sustaining treatment is not mandatory when "the provision of such treatment would be virtually futile in terms of the survival of the infant and the treatment itself under such circumstances would be inhumane" (at 14888). In Case III, the parents have the discretion to choose or not to choose the surgery. We suggest that parents make a reasonable choice in not choosing the Norwood procedure. The suffering and disabilities imposed by the treatment itself on an infant, with limited prospects for survival and a healthy life even with the procedure, justify their decision to refrain. At the same time, their choice of the procedure would be defensible. Parental desire to save their child from certain death gives support to their choice. The obligation to alleviate pain, suffering, and disability is as serious as an obligation to save an endangered life.

3.1   ENHANCING QUALITY OF LIFE

Medicine, throughout history, has contributed to quality of life by helping persons to maintain their health and by remedying the effects of illness. More recently, medical skills have been employed to improve on normal conditions: Cosmetic surgery responds to the desires of individuals for a more beautiful appearance, administration of growth hormone increases height for short-statured persons, and steroids augment athletic prowess. Genetic technologies offer the potential to improve physical and intellectual capacities. How do these enhancement capabilities fit the goals of medicine? Do they raise any special ethical problems for the clinician? Recent discussions of this issue often distinguish between treatment and enhancement. Treatments attempt to provide characteristics that are normal in the population to persons who lack them, for example, increase of stature to the mean height of the population, or increase of very small breasts to average size. These interventions are thought to conform more closely to the traditional goals of medicine. Enhancements augment already normal capacities above the normal range. Because the meaning of "normal" in these descriptions is ambiguous, it is difficult to draw a sharp distinction between these two capabilities of medicine.

Treatments do remain closer, however, to the usual procedures of medicine in that they are initiated because of a documented deficit, such as growth hormone deficiency. Enhancements, on the other hand, do not remedy a documented physical deficit but respond to the desire of the patient (or sometimes their surrogates, as when parents request growth hormone for their children who are genetically short-statured rather than growth hormone–deficient). Here the desire of the patient can have many motives, such as attaining competitive advantage, improving self-image and self-esteem, or feeling equal in one's peer group.

These forms of enhancement raise questions about their place within medicine. Medical indications are lacking and tenuous and, although done to respond to patient preference and to improve quality of life, they are particularly susceptible to contextual problems; that is, they may involve unfairness in distribution of resources (competitive advantage goes to those able to pay), complicity with suspect cultural norms (idealized body types), interference with social practices (fairness in athletic competition), fostering inauthenticity and false self-images, and the conversion of medicine into little more than a lucrative commercial activity for the enrichment of practitioners. Thus, although many enhancement practices have entered into the daily practice of medicine, such as cosmetic surgery or the prescription of sildenafil (Viagra), practitioners should be aware that many enhancement practices are on the fringe of the traditional goals of medicine and may have negative personal and social consequences. It is our opinion that interventions should respond not only to patient preferences and quality of life but also to medical indications based on demonstrable deficits in the health of the patient.

Special Section: In Pursuit of Perfect People: The Ethics of Enhancement. *Camb Q Healthc Ethics* 2000;9(3).

Special Supplement. Is Better Always Good? The Enhancement Project. *Hastings Cent Rep* 1998;28(1).

Parens E, ed. *Enhancing Human Traits: Conceptual Complexity and Ethical Implications*. Washington, DC: Georgetown University Press; 1998.

3.1.1 Dementia and Quality of Life

The occurrence of Alzheimer's disease or any other of the dementing diseases is a tragedy for patient and family. These medical conditions entail serious deterioration in the quality of life as perceived by the patient and as perceived by their families, friends, and health care providers. They pose difficult challenges to health care practitioners. Some of those challenges are ethical in nature: truthfully informing the patient of the diagnosis; imposing limits on lifestyle, such as driving; and deciding about living arrangements, use of restraints, and treatment at end of life. In recent years, improvements in the understanding of these conditions and in treatment of persons suffering from them have alleviated some burdens. In general, the ethical approach to such conditions calls for the least restrictive measures compatible with the safety and comfort of the patient. Other ethical problems may arise.

Case. Mr. R.P., an accomplished cabinet maker and a congenial, loving person, begins to show the characteristic signs of Alzheimer's disease (AD) at the age of 66 years. He slips rapidly into extreme forgetfulness and confusion, accompanied by outbreaks of anger, particularly at his wife of 40 years. His physician performs tests to exclude other possible causes. His sons, who are partners in his business, find it necessary to prevent him from coming to the factory and from entering his home workshop, which infuriates him. The family learns from a Web site about the drug donepezil, which has shown some efficacy in improving mental functioning. They request the physician to prescribe this drug for their father.

COMMENT. Although particular ethical quandaries are posed by patients with AD, the most general problem is the maintenance of their dignity, independence, sense of self-respect, and connectedness with their social and physical environment. These qualities are often seriously undermined by even well-meaning providers and by restrictive arrangements that often exacerbate the problems (e.g., restraints have been shown to accelerate physical and psychologic deterioration and increase sedative drug use). Many techniques have been devised to support the dignity of even badly affected patients and have been shown to improve their quality of life; thoughtful advice from knowledgeable providers can often help. Medication may have positive effects on some problems commonly associated with AD, such as depression, delusions, and psychoses. However, drug treatment to retard loss of function and improve lost functions is still in the early stages.

RECOMMENDATION. In Mr. R.P.'s case, use of donepezil may have some positive effect, because its efficacy appears to be greatest in the earlier stages of AD. Its efficacy is relatively brief, however, and the patient will return to progressive dementia. Thus, providers and family should seriously consider whether a transitory and slight improvement in mental status will truly improve the patient's quality of life. As the efficacy of the drug wanes, the patient will again slip into dementia, repeating the distressing experience of gradual loss of function. Also, this class of drugs (cholinesterase inhibitors) has unpleasant side effects, such as nausea, diarrhea, and insomnia, that might be particularly distressing to a person with diminished mental function. Thus, this medical intervention that, in principle, may be medically indicated, and is desired by the surrogates, may have a detrimental effect on the overall quality of life of the patient. Behavioral, environmental, and social interventions, and education for his family, are advisable. Drug treatment for AD is promising but at the present time must be employed with discretion.

Special Section: The Ethics of Alzheimer's Disease. *J Clin Ethics* 1998;9(1).

3.1.2 Rehabilitation

Rehabilitation medicine aims at an improvement in quality of life, demonstrated by restoration of mobility, ability to work, and independent living. The autonomy of the patient is a primary goal, and the preferences and values of the patient define the goal. The cooperation of the patient is crucial. In this setting, several special ethical problems predominate. These problems sometimes arise because the patient's preferences and judgment of personal quality of life conflict with the physiatrist's medical knowledge and values.

EXAMPLE. A program of rehabilitation is recommended to the gymnastics instructor described in Section 3.0.2. He initially refuses to participate in such a program, stating, "I'm crippled and the quality of my life is so bad that it can't be improved." The rehabilitation team has a different view of his possibilities. They invite him to continue to discuss the issues and propose some short-term goals.

COMMENT. This case could be discussed in Chapter 2, because it is an instance of problems arising around patient preferences. Quality of life is central, however, to the physiatrist's evaluation of whether the patient's wishes should be honored. Rehabilitation medicine stresses an educational framework for treatment: Persons are taught skills and taught to live within the limits of inevitable disabilities. Similarly, ethical problems regarding appropriate treatment should be first addressed as educational issues. The physician attempts to aid the patient to understand the problem in as full a context as possible.

Special Issue. Ethical and Policy Issues in Rehabilitation Medicine. *Hastings Cent Rep* 1987;17.

3.1.3 Relief of Pain and Suffering and Palliative Care

Relief of pain is a medical goal sought by medication, surgery, and rehabilitation, but pain is often only one component of the psychologic, social, and spiritual phenomenon usually called suffering. Concentration on the physiologic components of pain through pharmacologic or surgical interventions, without equal attention to the psychologic, social, and spiritual, may bring little relief. Even if relief is achieved in the physiologic sense, other important ethical responsibilities may be left unfulfilled, for example, aiding patients to deal with their death and its effect on others. Physicians should make themselves aware of these components and seek assistance from those expert in dealing with them. The presence of religious counselors is often of immeasurable value to the patient, to the family, and to the physician. Two problems commonly arise in palliative care: the problem of pain without evident physical cause and the palliation of care for the dying patient.

3.1.4 Treatment of Chronic Pain

Frequently, patients complain of pain without apparent physical cause. Care of these patients can be extraordinarily difficult.

Case. Mr. T.W., a 42-year-old insurance broker, visits his physician, complaining of severe, diffuse pain which, he said, had been "creeping up" on him for several months. Now, it is incessant, moves about the body, from upper back and shoulders to lower back and lower limbs. Standing for any length of time is excruciating. His physician does a thorough physical examination, prescribes several imaging tests, and, after negative results, recommends a neurology consultation, which is also unproductive. A variety of pain medications are prescribed, with little relief. Mr. T.W.'s pain continues to the point of disability. The physician finally tells him frankly, "We can't find anything wrong with you. Your pain is psychogenic; that is, it comes from the mind, not the body. You really should see a psychiatrist."

COMMENT. Chronic pain often poses a difficult medical problem, because the specific organic cause is frequently elusive. It also poses an ethical problem, because physicians, once they suspect a psychogenic origin, tend to dismiss the patient as a "somatizer." Patients often hear conclusions such as the doctor's response quoted previously as an accusation that their pain is unreal or imagined. Even when a significant psychogenic component to pain is present, the pain is real. Instead of dismissing the patient with such a remark, physicians should provide symptomatic relief and consult with experts in pain management and in physical medicine. Psychologic assistance should be recommended as assistance in coping with pain, rather than as a substitute for appropriate medical management. Should the patient request certification for workman's compensation, a physician who has taken these measures can honestly certify that the patient suffers debilitating pain, although it may not be possible to meet the medical criteria for workman's compensation.

3.1.5 Terminally Ill Patients

The quality of life of terminally ill patients is enhanced by palliative care that includes skilled application of pain-relieving drugs. Unfortunately, skilled use of pain-relieving drugs remains a rare talent in medical practice. This failure, however, is increasingly recognized, and several new approaches are promising. They include research on pain and suffering, improved teaching and training for physicians and residents, and the emergence of several specialty fields, including pain medicine and palliative care medicine. The hospice approach provides many techniques for palliative care and should always be considered for terminally ill patients.

Patients should not be kept on a drug regimen inadequate to control pain because of the ignorance of the physician or because of an ungrounded fear of addiction. Medical licensing boards in all states are extremely cautious about physicians' abuse of their authority to prescribe drugs and sometimes carry that caution to the point where their oversight inhibits appropriate medication for pain. Local medical societies, in collaboration with academic medical centers, should attempt to assist the licensing boards toward a balanced policy in this matter. Attempts to achieve adequate relief of pain have another side effect, namely, the clouding of the patient's consciousness and the hindering of the patient's communication with family and friends. This consequence may be distressing to patient and family and ethically troubling to physicians and nurses. In such situations no ethical principle will resolve the problem. Instead, sensitive attention to the patient's needs, together with skilled medical management, should lead as close as possible to the desired objective: maximum relief of pain with minimal diminution of consciousness and communication. Of course, if the patient is able to express preferences, these should be followed.

Efforts to relieve pain by opiates entail the risk of respiratory depression, leading to death (although this adverse effect is seldom realized). Yet, relief of pain is one of the major goals of medicine, and it often is heartily desired by the patient. On occasion, it is difficult to manage pain medication so that pain palliation and respiratory depression are balanced. In such situations, should maintenance of adequate respiratory status take precedence over pain relief? Relief of pain and maintenance of function are both goals of medicine. When the goal of prolonging life can no longer be attained, however, the relief of pain becomes the primary goal to be sought during the remaining time of the patient's life. Pain medications, like most drugs, entail risks, and in the face of imminent death, a dosage regimen with higher risks than would otherwise be tolerated is rational. An ethical principle, sometimes named the principle of double effect, is often used to analyze this clinical problem.

3.1.6 The Principle of Double Effect in Alleviating Pain

The principle of double effect recognizes that, occasionally, persons are faced with a decision that cannot be avoided and, in the circumstances, the decision will cause both desirable and undesirable effects. These effects are inextricably linked. One of those effects is intended by the agent and is ethically permissible (e.g., relief of pain is a benefit); the other is not intended by the agent and is ethically undesirable (e.g., risk of respiratory depression is a harm). Proponents of this argument state that an ethically permissible effect can be allowed, even if the ethically undesirable one will inevitably follow, when the following conditions are present:

(a) The action itself is ethically good or at least indifferent, that is, neither good nor evil in itself (in this case, the action is the administration of a drug, a morally indifferent act).

(b) The agent must intend the good effects, not the evil effects, even though these are foreseen (in this case, the intention is to relieve pain, not to compromise respiration).

(c) The morally objectionable effect cannot be a means to the morally permissible one (in this case, respiratory compromise is not the means to relief of pain).

In this argument, the major practical problem for the clinician lies with the second condition (b), because often the intention of the physician is mixed: to relieve pain and to hasten the dying process. If it can be said that the dosages administered are clinically rational, that is, no more drug is administered than is necessary for adequate pain relief, the intention to relieve pain seems primary and the action is ethical. If doses in excess of clinical necessity are given, the intention to hasten death seems primary. Respiratory depression is a possible side effect of appropriate dosages of morphine (i.e., sufficient to relieve pain). It is "unintended" in the sense that, if pain could be relieved by other means that would not have the effect, those means would be preferred. If this latter intention becomes primary, the action would be judged unethical. Roman Catholic medical ethics employs this argument to justify clinically appropriate pain medication for relief of pain, even if the unintended foreseen effect is the shortening of the patient's life.

Beauchamp TL, Childress JF. Intended effects vs. merely foreseen effects. In: *Principles of Biological Ethics*. 5th ed. New York: Oxford University Press; 2001:128–132.

Case I. Ms. Comfort suffers from carcinoma of the breast with lymphangitic spread to lungs and bony metastases. She requires increasing narcotic dosage for relief of pain. Her pulmonary function deteriorates so that her Po_2 is 45 and Pco_2 is 55 when she is pain-free. Ms. Comfort is now receiving two tablets of 15-mg slow-release morphine every 4 hours. She asks for further morphine. Her physician hesitates, fearing that further medication, given her already compromised respiratory ability, will cause Ms. Comfort's death. However, he orders 30 mg of oral morphine every 2 hours.

Case II. A 63-year-old terminally ill woman, with widely metastatic esophageal cancer and profound malnutrition, develops peritonitis from a leaking gastrostomy tube. Attempted surgical correction of the leak was unsuccessful, and she continued to have peritonitis with severe abdominal pain. The patient and her family decide to have a morphine drip for control of pain. The dose of morphine is titrated to the patient's pain and to maintain her ability to communicate with her family. She experiences some decrease in respiratory drive and mental alertness. Six days after the morphine drip was started, the patient is no longer responsive. Her husband asks whether the inevitable could not be hastened. The attending physician himself dials up the morphine to 20 mg/h. The patient lapses into coma. She dies 12 hours later.

COMMENT. The morphine drip is administered in response to pain with the knowledge that it increases the risk of respiratory depression. In Case I, the dosage is maintained at a level needed to achieve a pain-free state. This is an appropriate application of the principle of double effect. In Case II, the dosage, at first rational, was increased to a point at which death was clearly intended. In that case, the ethical problem of euthanasia is raised. This is discussed in Section 3.3, as is the related issue of "terminal sedation."

3.2 OBJECTIVE CRITERIA FOR QUALITY OF LIFE

Quality-of-life evaluations, whether personal or observer, are subjective in the sense that they reflect the personal beliefs, values, likes, and dislikes of the one making the judgment. The question is whether any objective criteria are present against which value judgments can be measured and/or about which all persons would agree. This is a philosophical question of great complexity. For the purposes of clinical judgment we assume that no definitive answer is available. We suggest, however, that broad, if not universal, agreement would be possible on the following descriptions:

(a) Restricted quality of life is an appropriate objective description of a situation in which a person suffers from severe deficits of physical or mental health; that is, the person's functional abilities depart from the normal range found in humans. This is a judgment that might be made by the one who lives the life or by others who observe that person. Clearly, as noted previously, the evaluation by the observer and by the one living the life may differ. So, Mr. Cope, the diabetic patient who has multiple medical problems, considers his life worthwhile, whereas observers may judge otherwise.

(b) Minimal quality of life is an appropriate objective description for the situation in which a patient or an observer (such as the physician or family member) views one whose general physical condition has greatly deteriorated, whose ability to communicate with others is severely restricted, and who suffers discomfort and pain.

EXAMPLE. A profoundly demented 85-year-old man is confined to bed with severe arthritis, persistent decubitus ulcers, and diminished respiratory capacity. He must be tube-fed and restrained, and he requires opiate analgesia for pain.

(c) Quality of life below minimal is an appropriate objective description of the situation in which the patient suffers extreme physical debilitation and complete and irreversible loss of sensory and intellectual activity. It might even be suggested that this state would be better described as having no quality, because the ability for personal evaluation has presumably been lost by the person in such a condition. This description applies to persons in a persistent vegetative state (Section 3.2.2).

COMMENT. It is our assumption that few persons would consider either of these latter conditions (b, c) to be good and that those in such conditions would not choose to be in them, if they were able to choose. Many persons, on contemplating these futures for themselves, might say, "I would rather be dead." This is a cautious assumption, because persons seem to judge differently when imagining a situation than they do when actually in such a situation. Still, we address here only the most extreme case, in which a person has permanently lost the ability to interact with the world and with persons. Further, we do not take this assumption alone as the basis for any decision that would lead to the death of the patient. The conditions explained in Chapters 1, 2, and 4 must also be weighed in making a decision about proportionate care (Section 3.2.4).

3.2.1 Minimal Quality of Life

Patients whose condition fits the criteria for minimal quality of life may require life-sustaining interventions. The ethical question is whether such a quality of life justifies support of continued life. Reference to (minimal) quality of life to justify refraining from life-sustaining interventions requires serious deliberation and discretion.

Case I. Mr. B.R. is an 84-year-old man living in a nursing home. He was diagnosed as having Alzheimer's dementia 5 years ago. He is chairbound and does not respond meaningfully to human attention, but is often very agitated. He cannot now express, nor has he previously expressed, preferences regarding care. He is otherwise physically healthy. He is difficult to feed, frequently choking and expelling food. He has been treated several times in the past month for aspiration pneumonia with antibiotics and fluids. During the night, he develops a violent cough and wheezing. He has a fever of 100°F. The visiting physician diagnoses aspiration pneumonia. Should he be treated again?

Case II. Mrs. A.W., a 34-year-old woman, married with three children, has had a long history of scleroderma and ischemic ulcerations of fingers and toes. She is admitted with renal failure. The big toe of her right foot and several fingers of her left hand became gangrenous. Several days later she consents to amputation of the right foot and the thumb and first finger of her left hand. After surgery, she is alternately obtunded and confused. She develops pneumonia and is placed on a respirator. The remaining fingers of her left hand become gangrenous, and more extensive amputation is required. Her renal condition worsens, and it is now necessary to consider initiating dialysis. The attending physician says, "How could anyone want to live a life of such terrible quality?" Should the respirator be discontinued? Should dialysis be initiated?

COMMENT. In Mr. B.R.'s case, quality of life refers to the observer's assessment in light of his low levels of physical and mental activity. Nothing is known about Mr. B.R.'s own subjective experience. Mr. B.R. will suffer recurring episodes of aspiration. Use of feeding tubes will probably entail restraints because of Mr. B.R.'s frequent agitation. Quality of life, then, has become a relevant consideration, but only insofar as it refers to an objective state, particularly, the inability to control motor activities and to cooperate with care in any way. Mr. B.R.'s chronologic age is not, in itself, a reason to refrain from treating; it becomes relevant only insofar as his chronologic age correlates with this physiologic state and with an increasingly less positive prognosis. This objective state makes achievement of medical goals increasingly impossible at the same time medical problems continue to arise. In this case, both considerations of probabilistic futility and quality of life are relevant. In Case II, the severe physical deficits and problems of rehabilitation faced by Mrs. A.W. evoke in the observer an assessment that "No one would want to live that way." This, of course, cannot be verified by Mrs. A.W. at this time. Mrs. A.W. has multiple problems, but all are potentially reversible, with the exception of the loss of extremities. In addition, she herself has consented to the initial amputations, suggesting her willingness to live with these deficits. Finally, her vital personality before her surgery suggested to the staff that she had the ability to cope with rehabilitation and the difficulties of subsequent life.

RECOMMENDATION. In our opinion, it is ethically permissible to refrain from treating Mr. B.R.'s pneumonia after several episodes have shown this to be the beginning of a recurring pattern. Thus, it is ethically permissible to refrain from treatment of pneumonia, permitting this disease to be, as it was once called, "the old man's friend." There is no obligation to proceed with measures, such as gastronomy or gastrogavage, that would require the insult of permanent constraint and increase the risk of infection. On the other hand, it is ethically obligatory to continue to treat Mrs. A.W.: Significant medical goals can still be attained and, although her current preferences cannot be ascertained, it can be presumed that she favors continued treatment.

3.2.2 Quality of Life Below Minimal

Quality-of-life discussions often take place in situations where an ethical decision must be made about continuing life-supporting interventions for a patient who is unable to express any personal preferences or whose expression is indiscernible or indecipherable as the result of mental incapacity. In addition, physicians may suspect that, if some suggested intervention succeeds, the patient will survive, but with severe deficits of physical and mental capacity. The question is then asked, "Is such a life worth living?" In this sense, raising the issue of quality of life seems equivalent to wondering whether no life at all is better than a life that meets the criteria for "below minimal." Although this is a difficult philosophical question, the pressure of clinical decisions demands a practical resolution; the following sections suggest some consideration appropriate to clinical decisions of this sort.

Weir R. *Abating Treatment with Critically Ill Patients.* New York: Oxford University Press; 1989.

Case. Mrs. Care, the patient with multiple sclerosis, is living at home. She has a respiratory arrest associated with gram-negative pneumonia and septicemia. She is rushed to the hospital and placed on a respirator. After 2 weeks, Mrs. Care has not recovered consciousness; a neurology consultant states that Mrs. Care has the neurological signs consistent with persistent vegetative state. At no time in the course of her care has she expressed any clear preferences about her future. Should respiratory support be continued?

COMMENT. (a) Mrs. Care is not dead in relation to brain function criteria. That is, she has not lost all higher and lower brain functions. She still has brainstem activity, respiration, and heartbeat. Thus, she is not legally dead (Section 1.5).

(b) Persistent vegetative state (PVS) is a neurologic diagnosis defined as "a sustained, complete loss of self-aware cognition with wake/sleep cycles and other autonomic functions remaining relatively intact. The condition can either follow acute, severe bilateral cerebral damage or develop gradually as the end stage of a progressive dementia." Studies show that, when properly diagnosed, recovery of consciousness is almost unprecedented. The majority of these patients will not require respiratory support but will require artificial nutrition. Because persons in PVS retain some reflex activities, they may have some eye movement, swallowing, grimacing, and pupillary adjustment to light. This is naturally quite disturbing to observers, leading them to hold out much more hope for recovery than is actually warranted by the clinical facts. Medical interventions promise no benefit beyond sustaining organic life.

(c) All the functions usual to human interaction and, to the best of the observer's knowledge, all forms of cognitive and sensory experience are absent or extremely deficient. It is highly unlikely that any of these functions will be recovered.

(d) Care must be taken not to mistake PVS for another neurologic condition known as "locked-in state." In this latter condition, lesions in the midbrain paralyze efferent pathways governing movement and communication but leave consciousness intact. Neurologic consultation is required to make the differential diagnosis.

Ashwal S, Cranford R. Medical aspects of the persistent vegetative state—a correction. The Multi-Society Task Force on PVS. *N Engl J Med* 1995;333(2):130.

COMMENT. Note how this version of the case differs from Mrs. Care's condition as described at Section 1.2.1, where her death is imminent. In that situation, the judgment that further intervention is futile in achieving medical goals justifies the decision to discontinue mechanical support. In this case, Mrs. Care is neither dead nor imminently dying. Her MS has not advanced to the point where it can be considered terminal; at this point, she may have a number of years of life ahead. If her pneumonia resolves and she can be weaned from the respirator, she will not recover from her underlying disease, nor will she return to mental functioning sufficient for communication. Her life, supported by mechanical means, will consist of vegetative activities alone (as far as can be known). On the other hand, if respirator support is removed, Mrs. Care may breathe on her own and continue to live in a persistent vegetative state. Life in a vegetative state seems to the physician and the family a life of lower than minimum—of no quality. Their hope is that, once the respirator is discontinued, Mrs. Care will die quickly.

RECOMMENDATION. In our judgment, it is ethically permissible to discontinue respiratory support and all other forms of life-sustaining treatment. We argue that the conjunction of four features of this case justifies such a decision:

(a) In the state of irreversible loss of cognitive and communicative function, the individual no longer has any "interests"; that is, nothing that happens to the patient can in any way advance his or her welfare nor can the individual evaluate any event or state that occurs. Thus, if no interests can be served, life-sustaining interventions are not mandatory.

(b) No goals of medicine other than support of organic life are being or will be accomplished. We do not believe that this goal, in and of itself, is an overriding and independent goal of medicine.

(c) None of the other goals of medicine can be attained and thus no other medical benefits accrue to the patient.

(d) No preferences of the patient are known that might contradict the assumption that she would wish organic life continued. The conjunction of these factors justifies the conclusion that physicians have no ethical obligation to continue life-sustaining interventions. Where no interests are served and no goals of medicine are obtainable, no duty exists.

Case (Continued). Mrs. Care is in a persistent vegetative state. She is not on a respirator. She now becomes anuric and is in renal failure. Should dialysis be initiated?

COMMENT. This version of the case involves an instance of not starting an intervention rather than stopping one already being used. Many interventions are initiated at times when their use is quite rational. The achievement of important goals is still seen as possible. When these goals cannot be achieved, and when there are other important considerations, for example, absence of patient preference and quality of life below the minimal, they may be discontinued. Some clinicians believe that there is an ethical difference between starting and stopping, the former being more permissible than the latter. There may be psychologic or emotional differences; some physicians find it more troubling to stop an ongoing intervention than not to initiate a new one. The initiation of treatment expresses some measure of hope and assuages the uncertainty that besets clinical medicine. If, despite the physician's efforts, the patient succumbs to the disease, the physician has tried and done her best. However, in withdrawing or stopping treatment, the physician may feel responsible (in a causal sense) for the events that follow, even though she bears no responsibility (in the sense of ethical or legal accountability) either for the disease process or for the patient's succumbing to the disease. Finally, after deciding to refrain from aggressive therapeutic efforts, new medical problems, such as infection or renal failure, sometimes tempt physicians to initiate therapeutic interventions to deal with these particular problems. This is, of course, irrational, unless the intervention has as its purpose another goal more appropriate to the situation, such as providing comfort to the dying patient.

RECOMMENDATION. The decision to forgo support is justified in both versions of Mrs. Care's case. It is the common position of medical ethicists, supported by many judicial decisions, that the distinction between stopping and starting is neither ethically nor legally relevant. It is our position that there is no significant ethical difference between stopping and starting if the essential considerations regarding medical indications, patient preference, and quality of life are the same.

3.2.3 Nutrition and Hydration

Mrs. Care has been started on intravenous fluids and nutrients. Is it permissible to discontinue these measures after she is judged to be in persistent vegetative state? Mr. B.R. has deteriorated mentally and now lies in a fetal position, showing no response to verbal or tactile stimuli. Should a feeding tube be employed? In both cases, death would ensue from starvation and dehydration unless artificial means are used. Is there any special obligation to use these measures that distinguishes them from respiratory support or medication?

Beauchamp TL, Childress JF. Sustenance technologies vs. medical technologies. In: *Principles of Biomedical Ethics.* 5th ed. New York: Oxford University Press; 2001:202–206.

COMMENT. There has been considerable debate on this issue. Some authors argue that feeding is so basic a human function and so symbolic of care that it constitutes "ordinary means" and should never be forgone. They also note that forgoing these techniques is a direct cause of death. They wonder about the social implications of a policy that would deprive the most helpless of basic human attention. Other ethicists judge that the burdens of continual life of pain, discomfort, immobility, dimmed consciousness, and loss of communication would not be desired by any human, and those burdens so overwhelm benefits of life that there is no obligation to assist in sustaining life. In addition, continued nutrition and hydration may have adverse consequences for the dying patient, such as the discomfort of fluid overload. Finally, it is generally agreed that deprivation of nutrients and hydration does not cause the distressing symptoms of starvation in the seriously debilitated patient. The circumstances that justify the decision to forgo feeding are: (1) No significant medical goal other than maintenance of organic life is possible;

(2) the patient is so mentally incapacitated that no preferences can be expressed now or in the future; (3) no prior preferences for continued sustenance in such a situation have been expressed; and (4) the patient's situation is such that no discomfort or pain will be experienced. Given the diversity of opinion, we judge that either position is ethically permissible but prefer the opinion that, like all other medical interventions, the ethical propriety of nutrition and hydration should be evaluated in light of the principle of proportionality, that is, the assessment of the ratio of burdens to benefits for the patient (Section 3.2.4).

RECOMMENDATION. It is ethically permissible to forgo nutrients and hydration in Mrs. Care's case. She is in a persistent vegetative state and, presumably, lacks all experience. She will not experience discomfort from starvation or dehydration. In Mr. B.R.'s case, opinion would be more divided. Some commentators might note that, while profoundly demented, he is still capable of experience; his continual moaning and restlessness indicate that he is uncomfortable. If, then, discontinuing nutrients and fluids would aggravate his distress, it should not be done. It is unlikely that severe pain or discomfort will follow the withdrawal of nutrient support in a patient so deteriorated, and it is likely that death will occur rather quickly. Thus, it is our opinion that nutrition and hydration may be discontinued. Mr. B.R. should be kept as comfortable as possible.

3.2.4 The Ethical Principle of Proportionate Care

The traditional discussions of the ethics of forgoing life-sustaining treatment have turned on certain distinctions, such as omission or commission, withholding or withdrawing, active or passive, and ordinary or extraordinary care. One still hears in clinical settings such remarks as, "Withholding treatment might be acceptable, but once it's started, we cannot withdraw," or "Would extubation be active or passive?" Most ethicists now consider these distinctions to be confused and confusing. They are little more than summary statements of elaborate and sometimes faulty arguments, rather than justifications. Unfortunately, these terms are often substitutes for careful attention to details and for analytic thinking. We recommend that decisions to forgo intervention not be based on invocation of these classic distinctions.

Beauchamp TL, Childress JF. *Principles of Biomedical Ethics.* 5th ed. New York: Oxford University Press; 2001;119–136.

In place of these distinctions, the **principle of proportionality** has recently been endorsed by many ethicists. This principle states that a medical treatment is ethically mandatory to the extent that it is likely to confer greater benefits than burdens upon the patient. It is an updated version of one of the distinctions mentioned in the previous paragraph, namely, "ordinary or extraordinary." In recent times, the original meaning of this distinction, which originated in Roman Catholic moral theology, has been obscured. Today it seems to refer to the elaborateness, rarity, or investigational nature of a procedure. Originally, it designated the relation or proportion between the expected benefits of treatment in relation to its burdens and disadvantages.

The principle of proportionality, then, expresses this traditional concept: The correct test of the ethical obligation to recommend or provide a medical intervention is the estimate of its promised benefit over its attendant burdens. This test may be applied even when the burden of omitting treatment is death of the patient (which, in fact, may often be seen by the patient as a benefit). Although benefit-burden ratios are intrinsic to all medical decision making, it is important to notice that the principle of proportionality endorses this form of reasoning even in life-death decisions, which had often been thought to exclude such calculation in favor of an absolute duty to preserve life. The principle of proportionality states that no such absolute duty exists; preservation of life is an obligation that binds only when life can be judged more a benefit than a burden by and for the patient.

The principle of proportionality clearly applies to the patient's preferences. Patients have the right to determine what they will accept as benefits and burdens. However, proportionality also applies to medical indications. Physicians must formulate in their own minds the benefit-burden ratio to recommend appropriate options to patients or to their surrogates. The most difficult application of proportionality occurs when surrogates apply this principle to reach decisions for irreversibly incapacitated individuals who have left no prior oral or written directive.

3.2.5 Legal Implications of Forgoing Life Support

The death of a patient resulting from a decision to discontinue medical intervention on the grounds of quality of life has legal implications. In the cases described in these sections, the patient could be kept alive, perhaps for some time, by continued use of the respirator, by dialysis, or by some other way. It is the absence of "quality" of that continued life that leads to the decision to cease intervention. In contrast, the cases of termination of treatment discussed in Chapter 1 involved persons whose death was imminent and for whom further intervention was unlikely to attain medical goals. The cases in Chapter 2 dealt with termination of treatment that a competent patient had declined. Cases of both types are not likely to generate legal problems unless someone, such as a relative or another physician, claims the judgment of medical futility was wrongly made or that the patient's preferences were ignored.

Cases where quality of life is the central issue are more legally problematic. A person who could be kept alive is allowed to die. In legal theory, this might be considered homicide (although the traditional definitions of homicide certainly did not envision the problems occasioned by modern medical technology). The physician might be accused of murder or criminal negligence, or named as an accomplice in the illegal decision of another if he or she accedes to or does not object to the discontinuing of life support by another. A number of legal cases touching these matters have been adjudicated. We summarize the judicial decisions at Section 3.2.6.

It is our opinion that physicians are acting within the law, as currently understood, when they recommend that life-supporting interventions be withheld or withdrawn, unless specific law to the contrary exists in any particular jurisdiction. The conditions required for this decision are: (1) It is virtually certain that further medical intervention will not attain any of the goals of medicine other than sustaining organic life; (2) the preferences of the patient are not known and cannot be expressed; (3) quality of life clearly falls below minimal; and (4) family are in accord. We hold this opinion because, despite the legal perplexities, most leading cases thus far adjudicated have affirmed the legal correctness of allowing the patient to die when these conditions are present. In addition, we consider it advisable for institutions to establish an appropriate review committee for cases that present problems (Section 4.11). Finally, institutions should request their legal counsels to prepare clear instructions for the medical staff in view of prevailing local law.

3.2.6 Judicial Decisions about Forgoing Life Support

The most important judicial decisions relevant to cases of this sort are summarized below. These summaries are brief and, given the legal complexities, are provided only to familiarize the reader with the names of the cases and the principal issues. Fuller description and the proper legal citations can be found in many places.

Meisel, A. *The Right to Die.* New York: Wiley; 1998, with annual supplements.

Current Opinions with Annotations of the Ethical and Judicial Council Of the American Medical Association. Chicago: AMA, issued annually.

The judicial decisions in this area can be divided into two categories: (1) those involving competent patients expressing a desire to have medical treatment terminated, and (2) those involving incompetent patients whose guardians wish to terminate treatment.

Competent Patients. A California appellate court determined in 1984 that the right of privacy granted by the California Constitution is broad enough to allow a competent patient to refuse all medical interventions, including those that, once removed, would hasten death (*Bartling v Superior Court,* 1984). The case involved a 70-year-old man suffering from multiple chronic conditions, including emphysema and a malignant tumor on his lung. The patient sought the removal of his ventilator; his hospital refused, concerned that the patient would die if the machine were removed. The court sided with the patient, holding that the right to have life support discontinued extends to both competent and comatose terminally ill patients.

In 1990, the United States Supreme Court stated that competent patients have a constitutionally protected interest in refusing medical treatment, extending the protections granted by the California court to the entire nation, although for a different reason (*Cruzan v Missouri Dep't of Health,* 1990). The Supreme Court said the right was based in the term "liberty" in the 14th Amendment, whereas the California court had based the right in the California Constitution's privacy clause. Regardless of the source of the right, the end result was the same: A competent patient's protected interest in refusing medical treatment was recognized. Although the Court noted that the State's interests in preserving life, preventing suicide, and protecting the interests of third parties and the integrity of the medical profession could overrule the patient's interests, this rarely occurs in cases involving competent patients. Some legal scholars believe that the right of a competent individual to refuse life-sustaining treatment is "virtually absolute." Court rulings, however, have supported refusal of treatment only when patients, although competent, are extremely compromised by illness or injury.

Incompetent Patients. The second category of cases involves patients who are incompetent, whether caused by being comatose, mentally retarded, or otherwise impaired. In the first landmark case, *In the Matter of Quinlan* (1976), the New Jersey Supreme Court held that a patient's right of privacy includes the right to refuse to be treated with a respirator that merely prolongs organic life when the patient is not likely to return to a "conscious and sapient condition." The plaintiffs, the parents of a young woman in a persistent vegetative state, sought a court order to remove the respirator prolonging their daughter's life. The court determined that a guardian may assert this right on behalf of a patient and that a physician's determination that the patient will not return to a "conscious and sapient condition," coupled with concurrence by a hospital ethics committee, shields the physician and the hospital from civil and criminal liability if the life support is withdrawn.

This view, which equated an incompetent patient's right to refuse treatment to that of a competent patient, endured until the mid-1980s in most jurisdictions. The decision in *Cruzan v Missouri Dept. of Health,* the first United States Supreme Court decision in the "right to die" cases, began to clarify the doctrine surrounding the issue. The parents of Nancy Cruzan, a patient in a persistent vegetative state, petitioned the Court to order the removal of artificial nutrition and hydration tubes from their daughter after the Missouri Supreme Court denied the order because of a failure to prove that Nancy would have wanted to refuse the treatment. The Court decided that food and hydration tubes, like respirators, are medical interventions that can be removed at the patient's request. In the case of incompetent patients, the Court held that states may set their own standards for the strength of evidence required to prove that the incompetent patient would have forgone the treatment had she been competent. Missouri had adopted the stringent "clear and convincing evidence" standard, which has been applied by New York in similar cases (*In the Matter of O'Connor* 1988). It is not clear whether an advance directive is required to meet this standard in Missouri, or whether an oral pronouncement of the patient's preferences would be enough, as has been held in New York (*In the Application of Eichner* 1979), the court ruled that an incompetent patient's statements made concerning respirators while the patient was competent were sufficient evidence of the patient's preferences to permit the removal of the patient's respirator. All other states have used lesser evidentiary standards, although the Cruzan case makes it clear that they are free to adopt the higher standard.

A more difficult decision is that involving an incompetent person whose preferences are unknown. These cases appear when patients have never been competent, such as individuals who have been severely retarded since birth, or when formerly competent individuals never expressed their preferences. The courts have taken two main approaches to this situation. Some courts allow the patient's guardian to make decisions for the patient, taking into account the patient's "personal value system" (*In the Matter of Jobes,* N.J. 1987). This situation presents a difficult ethical situation for the guardian, who might be tempted to interject his own values into the decision-making process. Currently, all but two states accept the decisions of close relatives in similar situations, and 12 states will accept close friends as proxies.

National Conference of State Legislators. *State Initiatives in Health Care: Policy Guide for State Legislators.* June, 1998.

The second approach to situations in which the preferences of the patient were never known is to adopt the "best interests" standard, meaning that the intervention can be withdrawn only if it promotes the welfare of the patient (see Section 3.0.3). In one such case, the Wisconsin Supreme Court held that it is never in the best interests of an incompetent patient to withdraw life-sustaining medical treatment, including nutrition and hydration, unless the patient is in a PVS state, has issued an advance directive, or has otherwise clearly stated her desires (*In the Matter of Edna Spahn,* Wisc. 1997). This case, however, has not been influential.

Usually, court intervention in such matters is unnecessary, and when physicians and family members are in agreement as to whether treatment should be withdrawn, some courts are reluctant to intervene and have authorized withdrawal of treatment without a court order. One recent Pennsylvania case held that a close family member of an incompetent patient may request that life support be withdrawn without a court order if two physicians diagnose the patient as being in an irreversible persistent vegetative state (*In re Fiori,* Penn. 1996).

3.2 P Life Supporting Interventions for Children

The decision to withdraw life support from a child is especially difficult. Generally, young children are not yet competent to express preferences with regard to life-supporting interventions, and parents will usually have the power to make medical decisions for their children, so long as these decisions are in the child's best interests. However, determining the course of action that is in the child's best interests is not always easy. Parents have a fundamental right to direct the upbringing of their children in such a way so as to be consistent with their values, and this right is generally thought to extend to medical decision making. In determining the course of action that is in the child's best interests, the expected benefits of a treatment must be balanced against a parent's right to control the child's medical care in accordance with the family's values and beliefs.

Because children are a vulnerable group, health care providers should strictly adhere to the principle of nonmaleficence, taking no actions that would harm the patient unnecessarily. Because the duty to protect the pediatric patient is stronger than with adult patients, some actions that are ethically permissible for adult patients may be ethically prohibited with respect to children. One decision in which the ethical dimensions of an action are affected by the age of the patient is that of whether to remove artificial food and hydration from a patient. With respect to adult patients, this decision is ethically tantamount to the withdrawal of respirators and can be done if in the patient's best interest. This is not the case for infants, however, as the provision of nutrition and hydration by caregivers is considered ordinary care. This is particularly true when the infant is being bottle or breast fed. Ethically, food and hydration should not be withheld from an infant except in rare circumstances in which there is no hope for recovery, and the infant seems to experience no distress from lack of nutrition and hydration. Legally, the Baby Doe regulations specifically prohibit the removal of nutrition and hydration from certain classes of infants, such as those who have been hospitalized since birth. In the rare case where the decision is made to withhold nutrition and hydration from an infant, providers whose personal values conflict with that decision should be given an opportunity to withdraw from the case.

3.3 EUTHANASIA AND ASSISTED SUICIDE

Some persons may reach the conclusion that the quality of their life is so diminished that life is no longer worth living. This conclusion may be the result of unrelieved pain or suffering, or because they consider the prospect of deterioration or loss of spouse or friends unacceptable, or because they judge their lives to be a burden on others. Persons who come to this conclusion are often terminally ill and under the care of a physician. They may request their physician to cause their death quickly and painlessly. In other cases, patients may be incapable of expressing such a desire to anyone, yet appear to be suffering so much that some other person, a friend, family member, or care provider, may feel compelled to end their apparent suffering by causing their death. The term "euthanasia" has long been used to describe situations of both types.

Beauchamp TL, Childress JF. Nonmaleficence. In: *Principles of Biomedical Ethics*. 5th ed. New York: Oxford University Press; 2001.

Special Section: Physician-Aided Death: The Escalating Debate. *Camb Q Healthcare Ethics* 1996;5(1).

The word "euthanasia," which literally means "good death," has been used in many different ways, resulting in considerable confusion. It was long used as a synonym for "mercy killing," that is, deliberately and directly killing a sufferer to relieve pain. More careful usage distinguished among "voluntary," "nonvoluntary," and "involuntary" euthanasia. Voluntary euthanasia describes situations in which the patient consciously and deliberately requested death. Nonvoluntary describes situations in which the patient was decisionally incapacitated and made no request. Involuntary describes situations in which the patients were killed against their wishes. These distinctions, while clarifying to some extent, also cause confusion. In recent years, involuntary euthanasia has been condemned by all commentators and nonvoluntary euthanasia, causing death without the expressed desire of the patient, has been condemned by most commentators. The debate now focuses on "voluntary euthanasia."

However, voluntary euthanasia is now understood either as "aid-in-dying," a situation in which a patient requests a physician to administer a lethal drug. "Physician-assisted suicide" describes a death that a competent person deliberately chooses and also causes by self-administration of a substance that a physician prescribes but does not administer. Because the choice of the patient is central to both concepts, the ethics of both situations could have been discussed in Chapter 2, Preferences of Patients, but since the patient's choice is commonly associated, in legal and ethical discussions, with diminished quality of life, we choose to discuss it here.

Case I. Mrs. Care is suffering from advanced MS. She is blind, bedbound, obtunded, and appears to be in constant pain. She has expressed no prior preferences about end-of-life care. Her husband asks the physician to end her suffering by ending her life. The physician administers a strong sedative, followed by an intravenous bolus of 120 mEq of potassium chloride.

Case II. Ms. Comfort is dying from widely disseminated cancer and is suffering intense and implacable pain because of bone metastases, even though she is receiving high doses of morphine. She remains conscious and alert. She begs her doctor "to put her to sleep forever." The physician administers 200 mg of morphine sulfate intravenously.

Case III. Ms. Comfort is in the same situation as in Case II, but requests her physician to prescribe a supply of barbiturates sufficient for her to end her life, to give her and her partner instructions about appropriate dosage and administration, and to be present when she herself takes the prescribed medication to end her life.

COMMENT. In all these cases, the physician supplies a means that will rapidly and definitively interrupt an organic process that is necessary to continued life. This fact distinguishes these cases from the cases in Sections 1.1.3, 2.5, and 3.1.6, where the physician stopped or did not provide some intervention for the support of failing vital processes on grounds of futility, the refusal of the patient, or profoundly diminished quality of life. In Cases I and II, the physician acts directly to kill the patient. Case I is nonvoluntary euthanasia; Case II is voluntary, but the administration of morphine cannot be justified by double effect reasoning.

In both cases, the physician's action is contrary to law in all American jurisdictions. Case III presents the problem of physician-assisted suicide.

3.3.1 Physician-Assisted Suicide

Until recently, the exact nature of the physician's assistance in hastening death was not carefully defined. It was assumed that the physician would either prescribe or administer a lethal drug. In more recent discussions, the physician's role has been more precisely defined by those who advocate legalization of the physician's participation. Administration of a lethal drug presumably constitutes an act of homicide. However, prescription of drugs that the patient can take at will removes the physician from direct participation. The decision and the action of ending life remain in the patient's control. The patient, then, commits suicide, which is not an illegal act (Section 3.4.2). The physician's participation by providing the means should, say advocates, be clearly excluded from statutes that prohibit aiding in suicide. Physician participation, these advocates claim, is in fact a proper medical duty of relief of pain. This description is called "physician-assisted suicide." It has increasingly become the favored way of presenting the issue.

3.3.2 Ethical Arguments about Physician-Assisted Suicide

The public, the medical community, and medical ethicists are divided about the ethical propriety of physician-assisted suicide. The opponents of assisted suicide use the following arguments:

(a) Prohibition of the direct taking of human life, except in self-defense or in the defense of others, has been a central tenet of the Judeo-Christian tradition. It has been equally strong in the secular ethic. An ancient maxim of the Western legal tradition states that even the consent of the victim is not a defense against homicide.

(b) Medical ethics has traditionally emphasized the saving and preservation of life and the improvement of its quality and has repudiated the direct taking of life. The Hippocratic oath states: "I will not administer a deadly poison to anyone when asked to do so nor suggest such a course." Contemporary organized medicine reaffirms this tradition. The Council on Ethical and Judicial Affairs of the AMA states: "Active euthanasia . . . is not a part of the practice of medicine with or without the consent of the patient." The American College of Physicians adds: ". . . even if legalized, such an action would violate the ethical standards of medical practice."

AMA Council on Ethical and Judicial Affairs, *Current Opinions,* 1989.

American College of Physicians Ethics Manual, 2nd ed. Philadelphia: American College of Physicians; 1989.

(c) The dedication of the medical profession to the welfare of patients and to the promotion of health might be seriously undermined in the eyes of the public and of patients by the complicity of physicians in the death of the very ill, even of those who request it. It is possible that subtle changes would enter into the relationship of patients and their physicians should such a practice become common.

(d) Requests for swift death are often made in circumstances of extreme distress, which may be alleviated by skillful pain management and other positive interventions such as those employed in hospice care.

(e) Even if initial toleration of physician-assisted suicide is limited to the voluntary situation, it is possible that, once established, the practice might become more acceptable for involuntary patients who "would have requested" if they had been able. Similarly, the availability of quick death may bring subtle coercion on persons who feel that their invalid state is a burden to others. Thus, even when effecting a swift death at the request of a suffering patient seems merciful and benevolent, the acceptance of the practice as ethical may bear the seeds of frightening social consequences. The "euthanasia" program initiated in Germany in the first half of the last century with the support of many benevolent physicians was first directed only to the incurably ill; it gradually expanded into genocide. This is the so-called slippery-slope argument, namely, that tolerance for a questionable practice on the grounds that it is harmless will lead gradually to the toleration of more harmful practices, either by accustoming people to the values involved in the questionable practice or by the logical extension of the argument.

Proponents of assisted suicide counter with the following arguments:

(a) The commonly invoked distinctions between "killing and allowing to die," "acting and refraining," and so on, are spurious; thus, termination of treatment and direct killing are morally the same and, if the former is permitted, the latter should be also.

(b) Autonomous individuals have moral authority over their lives and should be allowed the means to end them, including the assistance of those who can do so painlessly and efficiently.

(c) No person should be coerced into bearing burdens of pain and suffering, and those who relieve them of such burdens, at their request, are acting ethically, that is, out of compassion and respect for autonomy.

(d) Often the burdens of pain and disability are the result of the "success" of medical intervention that has extended life; those who have effected this result have an obligation to respect the patient's desire no longer to bear so unrewarding a result.

(e) The maxim of the Hippocratic oath is outdated, because medicine could never have anticipated the ability to extend dying that it has today.

The maxim should be interpreted as it is in the modern version, The Declaration of Geneva of the World Medical Association, "I will maintain the utmost respect for human life . . ."

(f) Some influential voices within the medical profession, which is generally opposed to active euthanasia, have recently expressed reasoned, carefully circumscribed support.

COMMENT. These arguments pro and con are vigorously debated by proponents and opponents of assisted suicide. During the 1990s, efforts were made, by legislation and by judicial decision, to make legal "physician-assisted suicide." Three states (Washington, California, and Oregon) submitted to their voters propositions to make legal the participation of physicians in causing the death of competent, terminally ill persons who request them to do so. In Washington and California, the proposition was narrowly defeated; in Oregon, the voters narrowly accepted this proposition which permitted "assisted suicide" as defined above. The United States Supreme Court has ruled that, while no constitutional right protects assisted suicide, states may legislate permissively (*Washington v Glucksberg and Vacco v Quill*, 1997). Thus, in Oregon, the one state that permits physician-assisted suicide, physicians may prescribe, but not administer a lethal drug for a competently requesting patient who is terminally ill. A 2-week waiting period between request and prescription is required, and psychiatric consult is required only when the physician suspects that the requesting patient suffers from mental illness. Although the Oregon law has survived several legal challenges, recently the US attorney general claimed that the Oregon law violates the federal Controlled Substances Act.

Even though assisted suicide may be legalized, physicians will have to make conscientious decisions about whether to provide assistance to patients to end their lives. The practice of physician-assisted suicide will require difficult decisions about what constitutes decisional capacity and terminal illness, and whether all means of relieving pain have been exhausted. In particular, legal authorization limited to only competent patients in terminal illness will leave questions about the patients in equally distressing circumstances who are unable to request or self-administer lethal medication and about persons who are not terminal but who anticipate slow death from degenerative disease.

A request for assistance in suicide should be met in the following manner:

(a) A physician who finds the arguments against assisted suicide persuasive must inform the patient that he or she cannot in conscience cooperate but then offer to discuss the issue in depth with the patient in hope of finding mutually acceptable options. If the patient continues to request assistance in suicide, the physician may offer to resign from the case or to provide only palliative care.

(b) A physician who is persuaded by the arguments favoring assisted suicide must recognize that assisting in suicide is illegal (except in the state of Oregon at the time of this writing). Different jurisdictions have somewhat differing laws and different ways of dealing with the issue, but, in general, assisting suicide is a criminal act. A physician may choose to take the risk of legal liability, but should do so in full knowledge of the possible consequences.

(c) If a physician chooses to take the legal risk, he or she should be confident that the patient has decisional capacity and is suffering from a condition that can realistically be characterized as terminal. Consultation on these matters is advisable.

(d) The physician should explore the issue with the patient very carefully and sympathetically. The patient's medical situation, options for treatment, alternatives to suicide, comfort care, relief of pain, social supports, values, and attitudes should be discussed. The discussion should take place over time and might include others, such as the patient's spouse and children, closest friends, and religious and ethical counselors.

3.3.2 P Infant Euthanasia

None of the arguments that favor physician-assisted suicide apply to infants or children, because those arguments depend on the express choice of the patient. However, decisions to forgo life-sustaining treatment can be ethically justified. When such a decision is made, an infant or child may continue to live for a period and may experience what appears to be distress and pain. This raises the question of whether it may be ethically permissible, even obligatory, to terminate the life of the infant immediately and directly, rather than tolerate a slow, painful death. A few authors see a compelling logic in this position. As a matter of practice, however, it is difficult to accept: The primary justification for euthanasia, namely, the voluntary consent of the patient, is absent; serious abuses might follow such toleration and the killing of infants runs counter to the instincts of most persons. Adequate management of pain can be accomplished and measures of comfort should be instituted.

3.3.3 Terminal Sedation

Recently, the term "terminal sedation" has been introduced into the discussion about appropriate care of terminally ill patients. Terminal sedation describes the practice of sedating a patient to unconsciousness to relieve severe physical symptoms attendant on dying, such as pain, shortness of breath, suffocation, seizures, and delirium, and then withdrawing other life-sustaining treatments, such as ventilatory support, dialysis, artificial nutrition, and hydration. No lethal dose of opiates or of muscle relaxants is administered. The patient will die of dehydration or of respiratory or cardiac failure. A dying patient may request this procedure, or the patient's surrogate may do so when the patient is decisionally incapacitated. Proponents of terminal sedation consider it an ethical and legal alternative to euthanasia, as an amalgam of palliative care and forgoing of life support. Critics of this practice claim that it is unethical, because it does not observe an important provision of the principle of double effect, namely, the physician may foresee death but not intend it as a result of the action. The essential intent of the practice is to relieve symptoms and suffering by making people unconscious and unable to eat or drink, so that they will die soon and inevitably.

COMMENT. We believe that terminal sedation is like euthanasia, insofar as it directly intends the death of the patient; it is unlike euthanasia insofar as an independent and justifiable decision to forgo life support has been made, and the sedating medication is not the agent of death. Thus, we consider it a morally controversial practice. If patients, family, and physicians choose terminal sedation, they should realize that it can easily be abused by evolving into the practice of "putting to sleep" patients who do not meet ethical criteria for a terminal condition or who are difficult to manage clinically.

EXAMPLE. An admitting medical resident offers relatives of an elderly, demented patient with metastatic disease "terminal sedation" at the time of admission for treatment of pneumonia. This is a crude and unethical initiation of patient care, although it may be suitable after a period of care and evaluation on the basis of the criteria mentioned in Section 3.2.2.

3.3.4 Legal Implications of Euthanasia

Deliberately causing the death of another, unless justified or excused, constitutes a criminal act, as does cooperating in the causing of another's death. Although suicide is not itself illegal, nearly all the states have specific statutes against assisting someone to commit suicide. Thus, the physician who administers or provides a lethal agent is liable to a criminal charge of homicide or assisting suicide. Decisions to allow persons who are terminally ill to die, discussed in the previous chapters and sections, are also examples of "causing" the death of another. However, the clinical decision that further medical care would provide no therapeutic benefit other than to prolong organic life relieves the physician of the legal duty to continue to intervene with medical measures. Similarly, a competent patient has the right to refuse life-supporting measures. These are clear and accepted defenses against criminal and civil charges. A decision to kill the patient by using some lethal agent, even when death is imminent, does not rest on a clinical judgment about the futility of medical care. It is a decision that can be made by persons without medical skills, and the lethal agent can be a bullet, an electric shock, or poison. The "compassionate" intent of the perpetrator is not a defense recognized by the law. Currently, the request of the victim, even if competent and uncoerced, is not a defense. In such situations, anyone who kills another human being can be charged with a criminal offense. Physicians and laypersons alike must stand before the law.

3.4 SUICIDE

Suicide is the deliberate taking of one's life. It is natural to assume that attempted or requested suicide in part reflects a personal belief that the quality of one's life has become unbearable. As an ethical problem, it could be discussed under patient preferences, Chapter 2. However, because the physician will often encounter the problem either at the end of the terminal illness of a patient, when life is of "poor quality," or in the emergency department, when preferences can only be inferred, it is discussed here.

3.4.1 Treatment of Suspected Suicides

Suspected suicides are frequently encountered in the emergency department. Even when the suspicion is supported by evidence, such as a history and a suicide note, it has been customary to provide all means necessary for resuscitation and care if there are solid medical grounds to expect recovery.

Case. Ms. D.W., a 24-year-old woman, is brought to the ED; she has deeply slashed her wrists and overdosed. She is obtunded. She has been brought in several times before and is known to have a psychiatric history of depression. On her last admission she screamed that next time she should be allowed to die.

RECOMMENDATION. Ms. D.W. should be treated. The customary practice of disregarding the suicide wish in the emergency department situation is ethically appropriate, even though it seems to contravene the autonomy of the person. The following comments are germane to this situation:

(a) The ethical basis for suicide prevention is the well-authenticated psychologic thesis that the suicide attempt is very often a "cry for help" rather than an unambivalent decision to end one's life. Frequently, the fact that the attempted suicide arrives in the ED suggests the act was ambivalently motivated. Many suicide attempts are halfway. The suicide attempt may not be an act of autonomy but rather be an act resulting from impaired capacity because of a mental or physical disease or emotional conflict.

(b) Suicide attempts are often undertaken in psychopathological conditions that are treatable or under social conditions that are transient. It is sometimes possible to anticipate these problems. Physicians have an ethical obligation to recognize the suicidal inclinations of patients whom they encounter in their practice and to make efforts to assist them personally or by referral to a trained counselor.

3.4.2 Suicide and Refusal of Treatment

It is sometimes asked whether refusal of treatment by a patient is equivalent to suicide. If it were, the physician might feel constrained to prevent suicide or to avoid complicity. Significant ethical differences exist between suicide and refusal of medical care. Following are examples of these differences:

(a) In refusal of care, persons do not take their lives; instead they do not permit another to help them survive. Persons who abhor the thought of suicide may say, "I do not want to kill myself. I only want to be allowed to die."

(b) In refusal of care, death is caused by the progress of a lethal disease which is not treated; in suicide, the immediate cause of death is a self-inflicted lethal act. In refusing lifesaving care, the patient does not set in motion the lethal cause. The patient's refusal authorizes the physician to refrain from therapy; the fatal condition is itself the cause of death.

(c) Even though suicide and refusal of treatment both result in death, the moral setting differs completely in intention, circumstances, motives, and desires.

(d) The Roman Catholic Church, which condemns suicide, does permit its adherents to refuse care, even should death result, when treatment offers little hope and is burdensome, painful, or costly ("extraordinary").

(e) Many judicial decisions and legal statutes now distinguish between legitimate refusal of care and suicide. Most Natural Death Acts explicitly state that death following a decision authorized by these acts cannot be considered suicide for purposes of denial of life insurance.

3.4.3 Legal Status of Suicide

Suicide was once a criminal act in the Anglo-American common law, but all sanctions for suicide (which formerly had included confiscation of the suicide's estate) were repealed in American jurisdictions in the first half of the twentieth century. Thus, suicide is not illegal, although various laws do support suicide prevention. Most jurisdictions retain legal sanctions against aiding and abetting suicides. These apply to anyone who, under current law, provides aid in dying or physician-assisted suicide. The state of Oregon alone, as of 2002, permits physician assistance in the death of a patient, limited to the prescribing of a lethal dose of medication.

Chapter 4

4.0 ▪ ▪ ▪ ▪ ▪ ▪ ▪ ▪ ▪ ▪ ▪ ▪ ▪

Contextual Features

This chapter reviews the fourth topic that is essential to the adequate description and resolution of a case in clinical ethics: the social, legal, economic, and institutional circumstances in which a particular case of patient care occurs. These circumstances are the context of the case and so we call the topic "contextual features." Physicians and patients have various responsibilities and obligations to the larger world in which their relationship takes place: They have families, live in social and political communities, and are employed by, or contract with, health care organizations.

The patient-physician encounter occurs in more complex institutional and economic structures than ever before. Only occasionally does the traditional private relationship exist in which a patient chooses and consults a physician in private practice and pays a fee out of pocket for service. More often, doctors today stand in multiple relationships with other physicians, nurses, allied health professionals, health care administrators, third-party payers, professional organizations, and state and federal agencies, in addition to patients and their families. Similarly, patients stand in relationships with family and friends, other health professionals, health care institutions, and third-party payers. Physicians and patients are also subject to the varying influence of community and professional standards, legal rules, governmental and institutional policies, research regulations, teaching concerns, economic considerations, religious beliefs, and other factors. What is the import of these multiple responsibilities on the relationship between patient and physician?

Further complicating factors include changes in health care organization and financing, laws affecting health care access, and computerized medical information, storage, and retrieval. Contextual factors, such as costs and reorganization of health care, have created conflicts of interest for physicians, who, in addition to serving their patient's needs, are increasingly required to be responsible for the utilization and costs of health care. This social burden often is, or is perceived to be, imposed at the expense of benefits to particular patients.

The context of care influences the ways in which ethical problems are viewed, analyzed, and resolved. The context of care is related to the clinical case in at least two ways: It establishes the limits and conditions in which decisions take place, and it is itself influenced by decisions made by and about the patient. In this chapter, we will discuss the ethical relevance of both of these aspects of the contextual features. Under the topic of contextual features, we discuss (1) the role of interested parties other than the patient, such as the patient's relatives; (2) physician confidentiality; (3) the economics of health care; (4) the allocation of scarce health resources; (5) the role of religion; (6) the role of the law; (7) clinical research; (8) clinical teaching; (9) occupational medicine; and (10) public health. We conclude with a discussion of ethics committees and ethics consultation.

In this book, contextual features are discussed only in relation to clinical cases. These issues can also be discussed in relation to social, economic, and health policy. Such discussions are essential to a modern ethics of medicine and health care. **Justice** is the ethical principle most relevant to these discussions. Justice concerns the fair and equitable distribution of burdens and benefits to the participants in social institutions. Justice also determines how the rights of various participants are realized within those social institutions. Thus, many of the particular clinical problems encountered by patients and physicians arise from inequities in the institutions of health care and of society at large. Reform of social and health policy in accord with the principles of justice is an ethical imperative. However, in this book, we remain at the clinical level, where providers of care meet particular patients and attempt to provide appropriate care. We advise those who wish to learn more about the ethics of health policy to consult such books as those noted below.

Morreim H. *Balancing Act: The New Medical Ethics of Medicine's New Economics.* Boston: Kluwer Academic Publishers; 1991.

Daniels N. *Just Medicine.* New York: Cambridge University Press; 1985.

4.0.1 Loyalty and the Multiple Responsibilities of Physicians

The ethics of medicine has traditionally directed the physician to attend primarily, even exclusively, to the needs of the patient. It is clearly unethical to do anything to a patient that will not benefit, and may even harm the patient, in order to benefit the physician or some other party. For example, a physician who performs diagnostic or therapeutic procedures that are not indicated, under pretense of caring for the patient but with the intent only of collecting a Medicaid fee, clearly acts unethically. At the same time, it has always been recognized that physicians, in some sense, also have certain responsibilities beyond their patients. In recent years, the absorption of the once very private relationship between physicians and patients into large organizations that employ or contract with physicians and that enroll and insure patients has added a new dimension to the physician's duties. Frequently, physicians take on contractual obligations with these organizations that directly affect the ways in which they care for their patients.

The ethical problem posed by multiple responsibilities arises when it is unclear how to determine which responsibilities have priority in a particular case or when it appears that duty to one's patient is in direct conflict with duties to others. The moral principle of **loyalty** is appropriate to these problems. Loyalty is a sustained commitment to the welfare of persons or to the success of an endeavor, requiring an investment of effort and sometimes even a subordination of self-interest. All persons have multiple loyalties—to family, to friends, to a religious faith, to a community, to a nation, to a cause—and usually these can be managed without conflict. At times, different loyalties will pull a person in opposite directions, and a choice must be made. The tradition of medical ethics, the expectation of the public, and the common law assign a high priority to the physician's loyalty to his or her patients; we will discuss the conditions that limit that loyalty in the following sections. Finally, the principles of justice and the fair distribution of burdens and benefits within a social order may put a constraint on the physician's loyalty to patients. When policies are fairly and justly developed for the distribution of some good, such as transplantable organs or medicines in epidemics, individual physicians are obliged to adhere to these rules even if such adherence compromises individual patient's interests.

Beauchamp TL, Childress JF. Patient-physician relationships. In: *Principles of Biomedical Ethics.* 5th ed. New York: Oxford University Press; 2001:283–287.

Beauchamp TL, Childress JF. Justice. In: *Principles of Biomedical Ethics.* 5th ed. New York: Oxford University Press; 2001:225–272.

4.0.2 Allegiance and Advocacy

Physicians owe allegiance to their patients; that is, they must respect their patients' preferences and privacy and respond to their health and informational needs. This allegiance is an expression of loyalty. It requires that physicians advocate for their patients' interests, such as access to the most appropriate care or the preservation of confidential information before the interests of parties outside the primary relationship. However, this allegiance, while a strong obligation, is not unlimited. We shall develop this point in each of the subsequent contextual features.

4.0.3 Fiduciary Duty

It is often said that physicians have, under law, a **fiduciary duty** to their patients. A fiduciary owes undivided loyalty to those served and must work for their benefit. Fiduciaries have specialized expertise and are held to high standards of honesty, confidentiality, and loyalty. Above all, fiduciaries must avoid financial conflicts of interest that could prejudice their clients' interests. Thus, physicians, lawyers, accountants, engineers, and architects are typically considered fiduciaries, from whom clients are entitled to expect such performance and may sue if they are disappointed.

Despite the fiduciary rhetoric, the concept is clouded in practice. Courts and legislatures tailor the fiduciary metaphor to meet the nuances of particular cases and patterns of social responsibilities. Law applies the concept to medicine principally in contexts of abandonment, confidentiality, informed consent, and disclosure of financial interests. Some economic conflicts are prohibited, but many exceptions exist. Neither malpractice law nor licensing rules invoke fiduciary standards. Many new contractual and organizational arrangements in health care put great strain on a concept that has limited applicability. Merely invoking the fiduciary nature of the relationship does not solve the ethical and legal problems posed by multiple responsibilities of physicians in the new context of health care.

4.0.4 Conflict of Interest

The term **conflict of interest** is often used to describe a situation in which a person might be motivated to perform actions that his or her professional role makes possible but that are at variance with the acknowledged duties of that role. The term applies most clearly to persons who hold political office and who can use the powers of office to enrich themselves. More recently, the concept has been applied to other professions, including medicine, where it poses significant ethical and legal problems.

Spece RG, Shimm DS, Buchanan AE. *Conflicts of Interest in Clinical Practice and Research.* New York: Oxford University Press; 1996.

Symposium on conflict of interest in health care. *Am J Law Med* 1995;21(2,3).

EXAMPLE I. A group of internists pool resources to invest in an imaging facility. The volume of business at that facility creates profits for them. The prospect of profit may influence their clinical judgments about the need for diagnostic imaging for their patients.

EXAMPLE II. A pharmaceutical company recruits a number of cardiologists in private practice to perform clinical studies of the antihypertensive effects of a new calcium-channel blocker. The company pays physicians a bonus for each patient who completes the study. The utilization review team discovers a substantial decline in the use of any of the other calcium-channel blockers listed in the hospital's formulary.

EXAMPLE III. A managed care organization (MCO) recruits physicians by offering a generous incentive program in which physicians can receive a bonus of up to 30% of their base salary, depending on their record of not using high-cost medical interventions, including hospitalization, to care for a group of capitated patients.

COMMENT. One common conflict of interest in which physicians find themselves involves the use of incentive programs by MCOs. Often, these programs reward physicians financially for keeping treatment costs low, as in Example III. Economic incentives of this magnitude may be unethical inducement and, at least, give the appearance of impropriety. The AMA has taken the position that physicians must "assure disclosure of any financial inducements that may tend to limit the diagnostic and therapeutic alternatives that are offered to patients or that tend to limit patients' overall access to care." The AMA's view is that physicians must only verify that the MCO is making such disclosures, not that the physician must disclose such arrangements to the patients. The current legal trend supports this view that MCOs, not physicians, have a duty to disclose the conflicts of interest arising from such incentive programs.

A conflict of interest is not in itself unethical. It is a situation in which an individual is provided the opportunity and motivation to act contrary to duty to gain personal benefit. Some conflicts of interest can be eliminated. For example, a law could forbid physicians from owning centers for self-referral. Other conflicts can be discouraged. For example, the AMA declaration that it is unethical for physicians to own centers for self-referral except when this is the only way to meet a social need creates a presumption that such a situation is suspect and requires strong and specific justification. Given the prevalence of conflicts of interest in the world of medicine and the heightened public concern about their impact, serious ethical and legal scrutiny and broad disclosure seem reasonable.

AMA Council on Ethical and Judicial Affairs. Conflicts of interest: Physicians ownership of medical facilities. *JAMA* 1992; 267:2366-2369. Current Opinions, 8.032.

4.1 ROLE OF INTERESTED PARTIES

Physicians have a moral and legal obligation to exercise special care to promote the interests of their patients. Patients have an interest in the competence and honesty of their physicians and an interest in the appropriate response to their health needs. Thus, the primary interested parties in a clinical relationship are the patient and the physician. However, many other parties may have some interest in that relationship and its outcome. Traditionally, families have such an interest, and physicians have recognized the legitimacy of that interest. The authority of the family to participate in decisions about their relative's care is explained in Section 2.7. In modern medical care, many other parties claim interest in the care of patients: hospital and managed care administrators, public health authorities, third-party payers, employers, litigants, lawyers, and so on. They may seek information, exercise oversight, establish policies that affect care decisions, and even attempt to dictate care. The justification of the legitimacy of these various claims is the ethical issue.

4.1.1 Physician's Duty to Self and Family

Every physician, like every human being, has certain moral duties to self and to those who constitute immediate family, such as spouse and children. Duties to self include adherence to one's values, cultivation of one's talents, and preservation of one's own health. Duties to family include especially stringent obligations to promote their welfare and protect them from harm. There may be situations when physicians are faced with performances of duties toward their patients that entail risk to themselves and, indirectly, to their family.

Case. Dr. O.S., a 36-year-old orthopedic surgeon in private practice, instructs his office staff to "screen" prospective patients, noting any characteristics that suggest they might be in a high-risk group for HIV infection. They are to inform such persons that Dr. S. is unable to accept new patients at this time. He also has an HIV test performed on all patients without their knowledge. He defends his actions by asserting his right, and the right of his wife and any future child, to protection from infection.

COMMENT. The duty to preserve health and protect family, with the corresponding right to do so, is legitimate, but it must be evaluated with respect to the nature, probability, and seriousness of the risks, alternative strategies, the infringement on others' rights, and the social consequences of various courses of action. The following comments apply in this matter:

(a) For health professionals in general, the danger of infection by contact with a patient is low, but not negligible. The risks for orthopedic surgeons, given the nature of their work, is probably somewhat greater than for other surgeons and considerably greater than for physicians who do not have regular contact with bodily fluids. Risk of infection is related to the potential for percutaneous exposure to blood. Hollow-bore needle sticks pose the greatest risk to health professionals, and thus nurses, phlebotomists, house officers, and medical students are the groups at greatest risk. After a hollow-bore needle stick, risk of HIV infection appears to be low—about 0.3% overall. Further, postexposure prophylaxis with azidothymidine effectively reduces the transmission rate, by 79% according to one study.

CDC case-control study of HIV seroconversion in health care workers after percutaneous exposure to HIV-infected blood. *MMWR* 1995;44:929–933.

(b) Various protective procedures have been devised that, if properly used, appear to be an effective barrier to infection.

(c) Medical tradition praises those who care for patients at risk to themselves. Medicine's public reputation rests in part on this tradition, and the public expects physicians to act in this way, so far as is reasonable.

(d) Toleration of the practice of excluding HIV-positive patients would lead to the exclusion of many persons in serious need of care and the exclusion of many who are incorrectly identified as infected.

(e) All major medical organizations have asserted the obligation of physicians to treat patients with HIV infection. The AMA Ethical and Judicial Council states, "A physician may not ethically refuse to treat a patient whose condition is within the physician's realm of competence . . . neither those who have the disease (AIDS) nor those who have been infected with the virus should be subject to discrimination based on fear or prejudice, least of all by members of the health care community."

AMA Ethical and Judicial Council Opinion 9.131, Council Report. Ethical issues in the growing AIDS crisis. *JAMA* 1988;259:1360–1361.

(f) In Dr. S.'s case, he is using methods that are inappropriate, inefficient, and unethical, even though he has the laudable motive of protecting himself, his wife, and family from infection. The "screen" depends on stereotypes and will not efficiently exclude infected patients. HIV testing without consent is clearly unethical and, in many jurisdictions, illegal. It is not inappropriate, however, to urge voluntary testing for patients who might pose risks. He should seek counseling about the most appropriate methods to protect against infection.

4.1.2 Family, Relatives, and Friends of the Patient

Patients are located in a social context of other persons with whom they have various sorts of relationships and interaction. These others are often interested in the medical problems of the patient and sometimes play an important role in the way care is provided. It is common in the specialty of family medicine to say, "The family is the patient." This phrase designates an important strategy of care, recognizing that in all illness, causal and curative factors can be found in the personal relationships that surround the patient. The good physician understands and works with those personal relationships as he or she works with the patient. The role of relatives as surrogate decisionmakers was discussed in Section 2.7. They may have other roles, such as providing emotional or living support, providing information, serving as interpreter of the patient's values, or paying the bills. They may sometimes question the course of care and seek to serve their own interests rather than the patient's. The moral cooperation of these others should be sought and encouraged; their moral roles and claims must occasionally be sorted out. The role of families is often defined quite differently in other cultures, and ethical problems will sometimes occur.

Case. A Japanese-American family brings their maternal grandmother to their primary care physician. Grandmother is 72 years old, came to the United States 10 years ago, and speaks no English. She complains of weakness, weight loss, nausea, and fever of several months' duration. Her grandson, a computer engineer, tells the doctor, "In case you find cancer, we prefer that she not be told. That is the way with our older people. But we do want her to have full treatment." Studies reveal acute lymphocytic leukemia (ALL) with renal failure, a condition that has a 5% chance for clinical response to aggressive and prolonged chemotherapy.

RECOMMENDATION. In Chapter 2, we stated our repudiation of paternalism and, at the same time, our wish to respect, as far as possible, cultural values. In this case, we recommend that the patient be informed, through a reliable translator, that she is very sick, that decisions must be made about her care, and then asked whether she wishes to make these decisions for herself or prefers to have them made by another. An authorized delegation of decisional authority instead of simple acceptance of the culture's purported customs is an appropriate compromise.

4.1.2 P The Family of a Child Patient

In pediatrics, families are of central importance. The authority of parents as decision makers in the care of a sick child is discussed in Section 2.7 P. The primary responsibility of parents must be the welfare of their child. The parents of an ill child, however, are often parents of other children and have multiple responsibilities. Decisions about treatment may have major implications for their other children and for the social and financial stability of the family. Often, parents will devote almost exclusive attention to the sick child but, on occasion, they ask themselves whether this is unfair to themselves and their other children.

Case. In Section 3.0.1 P, we have seen Monica, born with a major myelodysplasia. Her parents have three other children, aged 12, 8, and 4 years. The 8-year-old also has a neural tube defect of lesser severity but is hydrocephalic with a shunt and is somewhat retarded. The family gains its livelihood on a small, unproductive farm and lives at some distance from schools and medical facilities. They have been very devoted to the care and education of the 8-year-old and are fearful that the other two children are suffering from the attention given her. They now face the prospect of another handicapped child.

COMMENT. In the case at 3.0.1 P, we recommended that medical intervention for Monica could be omitted, in accordance with the parents' wishes. However, that counsel was offered in view of the prospects of a life of great pain and suffering for the patient. The welfare of this family and of the other children was not, in itself, the primary justification. Nevertheless, it is an additional consideration that, although not in itself decisive, adds to the moral justification of the decision. Still, we believe that any decision to allow a child to die should rest on medical indications and the quality of life of that child.

At Section 2.7.2 P, the problem of incompetent parents was noted. Physicians and nurses caring for the sick infant or child may form views of a family that prejudice their opinion about that family's ability to decide or care for their child. Cultural or socioeconomic features of the family may bias providers against taking the parents' wishes seriously. On occasion, the perceived problems may be very real—for example, when both mother and father are addicted to drugs and alcohol, live in substandard conditions, and so forth. In other cases, the perception might be quite inaccurate. For example, Monica's parents were "mountain people," whose lifestyle and appearance were foreign to the staff of the distant medical center. Yet, they were caring and competent parents who made great sacrifices for their children. Again, appearances may deceive in the other direction. Intelligent and achieving parents, in protecting their social and economic status, may act to the detriment of their child's best interests and, because of their appearance and manner, be tolerated by providers. Cultural customs, such as the Hmong practice of placing heated coins on a sick baby's body, may appear to providers as child abuse. When faced with such situations, providers must first ask themselves whether their judgments are affected by their own biases and ignorance. If problems are genuine and pose a threat to the infant or child in the home environment, educational means should be employed and, if they fail, legal action should be initiated through the child protective agency.

4.1.3 Indications for Genetic Testing and Diagnosis

The principal goals of medicine concern the detection of disease conditions and their causes, followed by appropriate therapy. Usually, this task of diagnosis begins from observation of signs and symptoms in a patient who comes to the physician for advice. However, the rapid development of molecular medicine has generated many tests for the detection of genetic mutations associated with disease. These tests are not usually done in a symptomatic patient to detect present disease; instead, they predict the possibility of future disease. Even a positive genetic test does not necessarily predict that the person who tests positive will develop the disease or, if they do, predict its seriousness. Many diseases known to have a genetic predisposition are currently not amenable to treatment or even to preventive measures. Also, genetic tests estimate the probability of future disease not only in the patient but also in the patient's kinship that shares the same genetic heritage. This explains why this section appears in Chapter 4 rather than Chapter 1: Genetic testing must always be considered within the family context. When a mutation is detected in one member of the family, the question of screening other members may arise. Many of these tests are in the earliest stage of development, although many of them are commercially available for clinical use. The availability of these tests poses many problems to clinicians; in particular, primary care physicians, lacking the detailed knowledge of the genetics and the nature of the tests, may be asked to order a genetic test by a patient anxious about hereditary disease.

Case. Mrs. Comfort, who was diagnosed with breast cancer at the age of 54 years, suspects a history of breast cancer in her family. She knows her aunt and her grandmother died of breast cancer. She asks her primary care physician whether she should be tested for hereditary breast cancer (mutations in two genes, *BRCA 1* and *BRCA 2*). She has two adult sisters, two daughters, aged 23 years and 15 years, and one granddaughter, aged 2 years. She wonders whether her daughters, grandchild, and sister should also be tested.

COMMENT. Primary care physicians may encounter cases such as this. Many tests are available on the market and can be ordered. These tests always contain materials that advise genetic counseling, for which a primary care physician may not be adequately trained. Considerations about the advisability of genetic tests should cover several points, which if the primary care physician cannot explain, should be referred to a medical geneticist or a genetic counselor:

1. The nature of the genetic disease associated with the mutation, that is, dominant or recessive, penetrability, variability, and the epidemiologic and clinical course of the disease.
2. The accuracy of the test: its sensitivity, specificity, and predictive value.
3. Implications for treatment or prevention of future disease.
4. Implications for one's genetic kinship.
5. Questions of confidentiality, insurance discrimination, and treatment availability and access.
6. The educated and informed preferences of the person requesting the test and of other persons affected by the results.

RECOMMENDATION. The test for *BRCA 1* and *BRCA 2* is indicated when a family pedigree suggests that breast cancer follows a pattern of autosomal dominant inheritance. Mrs. Comfort's sketchy information is not sufficient to confirm this. A more detailed pedigree would allow a medical geneticist to discern this pattern and, if it appears, would recommend genetic testing. If the patient tests positive for *BRCA 1* or *BRCA 2* mutations, testing of other genetically related women is advisable. Also, when nonsymptomatic persons test positive, an explanation of the probabilities of developing the disease is necessary; even those who test negative must be informed that, because this particular genetic mutation is only one of the causes of breast cancer, they are not free of risk. Preventive options, such as more frequent breast examination and mammography and, most drastically, prophylactic mastectomy, must be clearly explained. The testing of minor children poses particular difficulties, because it may seriously affect their view of themselves and the attitude of their parents toward their maturity. It is advisable to wait until they can make the decision themselves. Finally, it should not be assumed that Mrs. Comfort's siblings will be interested in being tested or in Mrs. Comfort's test results; this must be determined by appropriate inquiry. As molecular medicine advances, many complex ethical problems about obtaining and using genetic information will appear in daily medical practice.

4.2 PHYSICIAN CONFIDENTIALITY

The sensitive personal information that a patient discloses to a physician may be of interest to parties outside the medical relationship. That information is traditionally, ethically, and legally guarded by confidentiality. Physicians are obliged to refrain from divulging information obtained from patients and to take reasonable precautions to ensure that such information is not inappropriately divulged by others to whom it might be professionally known. The duty of medical confidentiality is an ancient one. The Hippocratic oath states, "what I may see or hear in or outside the course of treatment . . . which on no account must be spread abroad, I will keep to myself, holding such things shameful to speak about." Modern medical ethics bases this duty on respect for the autonomy of the patient, on the loyalty owed by the physician, and on the possibility that disregard of confidentiality would discourage patients from revealing useful diagnostic information and encourage others to use medical information to exploit patients.

Confidentiality may be treated rather carelessly in modern medical care. Providers may speak about patients in public places. Records are not well secured and are accessible to many persons, including some who are not health professionals. The greatest challenge to confidentiality in modern medical care results from technologic developments in information storage, retrieval, and access. Computerization of medical records enhances statistical information and facilitates administrative tasks. However, the availability of medical record information to interested third parties, such as employers, government agencies, payers, family members, and others, threatens patient or even physician control over sensitive information. For example, growing use of screening for genetic diseases, or susceptibility to them, produces information of interest, not only to patients and their physicians, but to the patient's relatives, employers, and insurers. Lack of consensus about how to regulate access to such information poses a continuing problem for health care institutions and policy makers.

State laws have been uneven in protecting confidentiality. Recent federal regulations attempting to create a comprehensive system defining the value, scope, and limits of confidentiality will not be enforced until 2003 (Health Insurance Portability and Accountability Act of 1996, HIPAA). These regulations, once enforced, will set a floor for medical privacy and leave the states free to enact measures that will more stringently protect a patient's privacy. Health plans, hospitals, clinics, and health departments must make a reasonable effort to limit the uses and disclosure of personally identifiable information to the minimum necessary to accomplish the purpose of the use or disclosure. In most cases, the patient's consent must be given before protected information can be disclosed. Patients also have the right to access their record and, in some cases, to amend the information. They are entitled to an accounting for disclosures from all entities that have received the patient's protected information. Finally, the burden of protecting the information is put on the institutions, which may be subject to civil and criminal fines for violations.

Although privacy is an important issue, efforts to protect it may conflict with other social needs, including the ability of health professionals to exchange information when caring for a patient, the right of parents to sensitive health information concerning their children, and the use of data for research, public health, or audit purposes. Implementation of protection may also be expensive. Physicians, then, who bear the responsibility to protect their patient's confidentiality, must become familiar with the regulations and policies, must be as vigilant as possible, and must advocate for better control of information and for better policy and law to safeguard it.

Beauchamp TL, Childress JF. Professional-patient relationships. In: *Principles of Biomedical Ethics.* 5th ed. New York: Oxford University Press; 2001:303-312.

Department of Health and Human Services. *Standards for Privacy of Individually Identifiable Health Information: Final Rule.* 45 CFR Parts 160 and 164:2001.

Confidentiality is a stringent but not unlimited, ethical obligation. The ethical issue, then, is determining what principles and circumstances justify exception to the rule. The ethical justifications for limiting confidentiality are based on the principle of justice and depend upon the contextual features of the case. In general, two grounds for exception exist: concern for the safety of other specific persons and concern for public welfare. Both involve the possibility that other parties will be unjustly harmed.

4.2.1 Confidentiality and Protection of Other Persons

Confidential information may be divulged to appropriate persons when a physician is aware that lack of that information places some identifiable person at high risk of serious harm.

Case I. A 61-year-old man is diagnosed with metastatic cancer of the prostate. He refuses hormonal therapy and chemotherapy. He commands his physician not to inform his wife and says he does not intend to tell her himself. The next day, the wife calls to inquire about her husband's health.

Case II. A 32-year-old man is diagnosed presymptomatically with Huntington's disease. This is an autosomal dominant genetic disease (50% chance of transmitting the gene and the disease to offspring). He tells his physician that he does not want his wife, whom he has recently married, to know. The physician knows that the wife is eager to have children.

Case III. A 27-year-old gay man is diagnosed as HIV-positive. He tells his physician that he cannot face the prospect that his partner will learn of the infection.

Case IV. A woman arrives at the emergency department with serious contusions on the right side of her face and two teeth missing. Her nose appears to be broken. Her husband accompanies her. He explains that she tripped on the carpet and fell down a flight of stairs. She affirms his story. The ED resident suspects spousal abuse. He does not know the couple, however, and judges by their dress and manner that they appear to be respectable citizens.

RECOMMENDATION. In Case I, the physician should not divulge the husband's diagnosis. While the wife has a moral right to know of her husband's condition, which will certainly affect her deeply, it is her husband's obligation to inform her. The physician, while feeling distressed about the situation, cannot justify disclosure, because his obligation to respect his patient's preferences outweighs possible harm to the wife from not knowing her husband's diagnosis. The physician should encourage the husband to reveal his condition but should not himself divulge the diagnosis to his wife. In Case II, a stronger rationale is present for divulging the diagnosis to the patient's wife, namely, the possibility of harm to future children. However, serious efforts should be made to convince the husband to seek genetic counseling and to urge him to discuss the matter with his wife. If the wife is also a patient, the physician may encourage her to talk seriously with her husband about his health and their plans for children. Risk of harm to future children is high (50%), but that risk is statistical and might not occur. No assurance is provided that disclosure of the husband's condition will protect any given individual. Still, the risk of harm to the marriage and, possibly, to future children favors disclosure as a last resort. In Case III, the physician has a duty to ensure that the lover is informed of his serious risk, first by urging the patient to do so and, if this fails, by taking the steps prescribed in public health law and practice regarding contact tracing and notification.

Provisions of local law should be consulted. In Case IV, the resident should make the required report to authorities. State laws usually do not give physicians the discretion not to report. It is the duty of authorized investigators to determine whether abuse has occurred. An ED resident should be familiar with the characteristic physical signs of abuse that can frequently be distinguished from other accidental trauma. The apparent respectability of the parties is irrelevant.

4.2.2 Legal Implications

In a precedent-setting case, *Tarasoff v Regents* of the University of California (Cal. 1976), a college student informed his psychotherapist that he intended to kill a woman who had rejected his attentions. This threat was not communicated to the woman, whom the student subsequently murdered. The court ruled that the psychotherapist had a positive duty to take reasonable steps to protect third parties from harm, stating "the protective privilege (of confidentiality) ends where the public peril begins." The serious danger of violence to an identifiable person was a consideration that, in the opinion of the court, overrode the obligation to preserve confidential information obtained in the course of therapy. It is unclear how this decision would apply to other practitioners who obtain similar information in the course of providing general medical care. Further, not all jurisdictions accept the Tarasoff rule. Faced with such a situation, a physician would be wise to seek an ethics consultation and legal advice.

4.2.3 Confidentiality and Public Welfare

Certain information obtained from patients may suggest that the patient might endanger others but without identifying specific persons or occasions. Traditionally, certain communicable diseases have belonged in this category, and laws have been enacted that require physicians to report cases of communicable disease to health authorities. Many jurisdictions require reporting of health defects, such as seizures and cardiac diseases, that might render operators of vehicles dangerous to others. Where reporting laws do not exist, and often even where they do, ethical problems may arise.

Case I. Mr. Cure, with bacterial meningitis, refuses therapy and insists on returning to his college dormitory room.

Case II. A 28-year-old man who has been under a physician's care for severe peptic ulcer impresses his doctor as somewhat bizarre in attitude and behavior. He suspects that his patient suffers from a psychotic disorder and asks him whether he is seeing a psychiatrist. He calmly responds that he was once under treatment for schizophrenia but has been well for years. Then, in the course of an office visit, he casually states that he would like to see all politicians dead and was going to attend a forthcoming political rally "to see what he could do." Should the physician report the patient to the police?

Case III. A 27-year-old nurse in a dialysis unit is hepatitis B antigen–positive. She is reluctant to inform her social contacts and resists any restriction of her professional activities. She approaches a private practitioner for advice. She insists on confidentiality and after being advised to tell the relevant parties, including the hospital's infection control team, states that she does not intend to do so. Should the practitioner take steps to ensure that her social contacts are informed? Should the practitioner take steps to have her professional activities restricted?

COMMENT. In Case I, bacterial meningitis is an infectious disease. If it is listed as a reportable communicable disease, the physician should report it. Because the final diagnosis is not clear and could be meningococcal meningitis, which is contagious, the physician has the duty to communicate the information to college authorities and recommend that Mr. Cure be isolated in the college infirmary during the course of his illness. In Case II, the danger to others is less clear. No victim is identified, and the likelihood of violence is uncertain. The threat is vague and, as is often the case, possibly empty. This patient is obviously in need of psychiatric treatment and should be persuaded to seek it. The consequences to the patient of a police report might be significant. The consequences of reporting "suspicious persons" on the basis of suspicions aroused in medical care might also be socially undesirable. The index for reportable suspicion, in the absence of evidence, should be high. In Case III, the nurse may infect others and the possibilities for contact are extensive and difficult to limit. She is capable of arranging her social contacts so as to avoid infecting others. With regard to her professional life, she has a direct obligation to protect her patients from harm. If she refuses to do this by reporting herself and by restricting her activities voluntarily, the physician has a duty to report her to the hospital authorities.

4.2.4 Legal Implications

Most jurisdictions have statutes requiring physicians to report cases of certain types, such as sexually transmitted diseases, gunshot and knife wounds, and suspected child, partner, and elder abuse. The purpose of these statutes is to protect public health and safety, and their ethical justification arises from obligations of social justice. These statutes should be obeyed when the physician believes the legal criteria for making a report are met.

In recent years, many jurisdictions have legislated about the confidentiality of HIV testing. The legislation is intended to protect HIV-positive persons from the prejudice that often is directed at them when their condition is known. Usually, this legislation does not permit the testing of persons without their explicit consent and requires their consent to share the results with any other party. Exceptions usually allow other health professionals caring for the patient access to the results and permit health officers access to the information for the protection of others. A few states have passed laws that give physicians the discretion whether to notify sexual partners of HIV-positive persons. Physicians should be aware of the exact provisions of this legislation in their area.

4.3 THE ECONOMICS OF HEALTH CARE

Costs are incurred whenever medical care is provided. Those costs are paid by patients, by their families, or by public or private insurers, or they are subsidized by institutions or individuals. Patients and physicians have always considered costs in reaching medical care decisions. In the past, it was assumed that patients would pay the costs of their care and that those who could not pay would be subsidized by the state or the charity of physicians or institutions. The introduction of private and public forms of health insurance changed the economics of health care. More recently, social and political efforts to restrain the growth of health costs have had significant impact on the financing of care. Regulatory efforts, such as capitated prospective reimbursement, and market forces, such as for-profit hospital corporations and MCOs, are used as mechanisms for constraining costs. The ethical question is how the financing of care, and in particular, the cost-containment methods used by these new mechanisms, should influence individual medical decisions. How should the legitimate interests of third parties—health care institutions, insurance companies, labor unions, corporations, and government—be factored into clinical decisions about appropriate care?

Some physicians say that these interests should not be factored in and that their only allegiance is to individual patients; societal or institutional costs are not relevant to clinical decisions. Whatever is required by medical indications and personal preferences should be provided. This view is sometimes called the "professional model." Implicit in the professional model are two ethical assumptions: (1) Any departure from absolute patient advocacy is a breach of ethical duty, and (2) medical recommendations that are based on clinical judgments are "value-free" scientific decisions in which economic incentives play no role. We disagree with both assumptions. We disagree with the first because physicians face conflicts of interest under any economic arrangement and have incentives either to do too much, as in fee-for-service systems, or too little, as in managed care. We disagree with the second assumption because the variations in health care practice show how supply often drives physician decisions.

An alternative viewpoint, sometimes called "the economic model," proposes that physicians consider not only the benefits and safety of an intervention and the patient's preferences, but also its cost efficiency. This economic model suggests that physicians have both individual and collective responsibility to use limited resources so that fair and efficient care can be provided to all who need it. In this view, clinical judgments should also be microallocation decisions that are based ideally on outcome data about cost effectiveness and on the marginal benefits of an intervention. This view implies that certain patients, despite their preferences, may not get every potentially beneficial diagnostic or therapeutic intervention. In our view, the economic model represents an ethical approach to the conditions of modern medicine; its attention to effectiveness of intervention often serves patients well, and its focus on cost promotes a just system that benefits all. Still, it must be applied with caution, lest it become nothing more than a budgeting device for health care institutions.

4.3.1 Costs to Individuals

Some individuals are not covered by public or private health insurance. Many such persons have restricted access to care and probably have poor outcomes in certain chronic diseases. Other persons can pay for their own care; in the market system that prevails in American health care. Such persons have the opportunities to purchase such care as they desire or the type of health insurance coverage that provides for their needs. This does create some inequity in the allocation of care, because it may siphon dollars and professional talent into forms of medical and surgical care that are luxuries rather than necessities. A solution to these problems of social inequity will require a restructuring of the systems for medical delivery and finance. This is a policy and a justice issue. Still, physicians face an ethical problem when they attempt to decide whether they will accept the limited reimbursement from some insurors or restrict their practices largely to the well-insured patient.

4.3.2 Access to Emergency Care and Critical Care

Persons who require immediate care for a life-threatening condition may see a physician or go to the emergency department of a hospital. Some critically ill persons may be uninsured and unable to pay for the care they need. It is an ancient tenet of medical ethics that physicians should provide services in such situations. The Hippocratic writings state, "If there is an opportunity to serve a stranger in financial straits, give full assistance . . . love of humankind and love of the medical art go together" (Precepts VI.). Most emergency care takes place in hospitals. These institutions operate under various legal requirements that mandate emergency care in certain situations. For example, emergency departments are not permitted by a federal law (The Emergency Treatment and Active Labor Act, EMTALA) to transfer to other institutions any patient who is brought in or comes in with acute symptoms of sufficient severity such that absence of immediate medical attention might lead to serious impairment. This applies also to women who are in active labor. Transfer to another institution is permitted only after such patients are stable, that is, have received treatment necessary to ensure that no deterioration is likely during transfer or, for women in labor, have delivered. Despite this legal restriction, hospitals may attempt to reduce the financial burden of uncompensated care. Policies developed for this purpose may affect the decisions of physicians working in the institution.

Case I. A 28-year-old man was brought to the ED of a rural hospital after an automobile accident in which he suffered head trauma. He was unconscious, and his wife, who was not severely injured, informed the admitting nurse that they had no insurance. Evaluation revealed a transtentorial herniation and an acute subdural hematoma. The patient was treated with dexamethasone, mannitol, and phenytoin. Because the rural hospital was not capable of providing neurosurgery, an attempt was made to transfer the patient to University Hospital. When it became clear to University Hospital that the patient lacked medical insurance, the transfer was delayed, and the patient died en route to a more distant tertiary care facility.

Case II. Metropolitan Hospital is located in an urban area where crime and drug use are rampant. Its neurosurgery service is always busy. A large percentage of its patients are uninsured because, in that state, Medicaid eligibility criteria are high. Other sources of funds for indigent patients are stretched thin. Still, Metropolitan defines its primary mission as service to its local population, including those who are medically indigent. Although it accepts emergency patients from outlying areas, it requires proof from distant transfers of ability to pay.

RECOMMENDATION. Physicians who work in institutions that receive emergency patients have an ethical obligation to ensure that the traditional medical ethic of service to those in urgent need of care can be fulfilled in their institution. The medical staff should attempt to influence hospital policies to this effect. Transfer policies and decisions made in the emergency room must be based on medical indications rather than on financial implications of service in the particular case. It is legitimate for institutions to establish policies that limit the indigent care they provide, but these policies themselves should be consistent with ethical standards and the law. In Case I, the patient's medical indications, requiring immediate neurosurgical intervention, should have met with a prompt response from University Hospital. The solvency of the institution was not at stake. In Case II, the institution attempted to establish a just policy on the basis of a definition of mission in relationship to its prospects for financial solvency.

Case III. Mr. R.W., a 61-year-old construction worker who has health insurance through his union, was transferred from a rural hospital to a tertiary care urban hospital with a diagnosis of acute respiratory distress syndrome secondary to *Klebsiella* pneumonia. On admission, he was comatose and in shock. After 4 weeks in the intensive care unit (ICU), during which he developed many complications, including empyema and a cardiac arrest, he was weaned from the respirator. He was transferred from the ICU to a regular floor. He recovered without permanent end-organ damage and with good cognitive function. At discharge, his bill was $368,260. On three occasions during his stay in the ICU, the insurance company's case manager asked the attending physician whether outcome data was available to justify continuing the expensive tertiary care.

COMMENT. A serious review of medical goals is indicated when tensions occur between providing lifesaving care that is based on medical indications and patient preferences (expressed or presumed) and cost-effective care that is based solely on economic considerations. If that review confirms the probable utility of treatment, it should be continued. Physicians and payers must realize that any health insurance system involves pooling risk and is designed to achieve a balance between cases that lose money and those in which the insurance company makes money. The case manager was questioning whether the patient was likely to benefit from the costly interventions. In situations of very high cost, such as this one, the question was reasonable and should encourage physicians to examine whether they are using cost-effective measures, while, at the same time, aiming at the goals of medical intervention.

4.3.3 Managed Care

In the past decade, new financial arrangements have appeared in medical practice designed to control rising health care costs. Among these are various forms of "managed care" (MC), that is, organizations that integrate the financing and delivery of health care by contracting with health care professionals and hospitals to provide care to an enrolled population for a fixed annual or monthly premium. This arrangement describes the original form of managed care, the health maintenance organizations (HMOs), but other forms of MC include preferred-provider organizations (PPOs) and point-of-service (POS), in which patients under a managed care plan may pay extra for access to providers outside the plan. The percent of people with employer-sponsored health coverage who are enrolled in MC plans increased from 29% in 1988 to 73% in 1995. The percent of physicians who had signed contracts with MC organizations increased from 61% in 1988 to 75% in 1993.

HMOs are one form of MC arrangement. Many of these HMOs are for-profit commercial enterprises. The overall income paid by subscribers to the plan is used to pay the expenses of care, administrative costs, and dividends for shareholders. Usually, the physician providers share financial risk for caring for patients. In some plans, physician compensation may vary based on the physician's use of health resources in caring for a panel of patients. Thus, an incentive exists for physicians to be cost-conscious, to stress prevention, and even, at times, to balance the patient's needs against the physician's financial incentives. Managed care organizations establish cost-containment measures, such as selecting the population of potential members, setting rates and kinds of service, achieving economies of scale in facilities, and using prospective or retrospective utilization review of physicians' clinical practices. Some cost-containment measures directly affect the clinical decisions of physicians working in these settings: Physicians may be encouraged to make clinical decisions about particular patients that are, on the whole, both cost-effective and medically appropriate. This may take the unobjectionable form of merely advising physicians to be "cost-conscious," or take the more problematic form of providing incentives, such as bonuses or increased portions of the savings accrued, for physicians who reduce costs. Primary among the cost-containment measures is "gatekeeping," namely, the practice of assigning patients to a primary care physician who "manages" their care by selecting the medically appropriate and cost-effective use of procedures, specialty referrals, and hospitalizations. When the role of gatekeeper is combined with financial incentives for underutilizing health resources, the physician is in a potential conflict of interest situation.

Managed Care Ethics. *Arch Intern Med* 1996;156(special issue).

By 2002, the managed care system in the United States was a decade old. From a system in which costs were controlled by tightly managing the process of care and the range of patient choices, it has evolved into a less restrictive form of health care in which subscribers are generally free to choose their own primary care provider, to consult with some specialists of their choice, such as gynecologists, and to seek care outside the plan for a higher premium. Thus, the term "managed care" may now mean only that negotiations and contracts between employers, insurers, and providers have become the standard mechanism for setting prices for service.

In the earlier forms of MC, physicians faced many serious ethical problems related to rigid constraints on their clinical decisions and from incentive systems that favored reduction of costs at the price of quality care. At present, many of these problems have been ameliorated. However, the general ethical status of physicians who are either employed by or are under contract to one or many managed care systems deserves consideration.

4.3.4 Ethically Acceptable Contracts for Physicians

Physicians employed by or under contract to managed care systems should assure themselves that they can work within these systems without compromising ethical and professional standards. They should be satisfied that the conditions of their contracts consider the following issues:

(a) Quality of Care. When joining a health care organization, physicians must be confident that the organization has the resources, commitment, and ability to provide reasonable health care to its members. A specific definition of "reasonable" will vary with respect to local needs, practice, and resources. Physicians should ascertain whether the plan's constraints on the availability of resources reflect sound methods of technology assessment and criteria for quality of care.

(b) Patient Choice. Physicians should assure themselves that they can support patient's choices. These choices include (1) the right of patients to select their primary care physician (who should serve as their advocate rather than as their "gatekeeper"); (2) the right to select a specialist, such as an obstetrician or cardiologist; (3) the right to go to an emergency department without prior approval; and (4) most importantly, the right, on the basis of the legal and ethical doctrine of informed consent, to make their own health care decisions.

(c) Advocacy. Physicians should be assured that they may act as advocates for their patients in obtaining needed services. Although such advocacy should be based on sound clinical judgment, it should not be restrained by a climate of sanctions against physicians who urge compassionate consideration of individual cases that may conflict with the organization's policy.

(d) Full Disclosure. For patients to be allowed to make reasonable choices, they must be provided with adequate and truthful information. This includes information about their illness and the various options for treating it, even if some of these options are not available through the patient's plan. It also includes disclosure about the physician's financial incentives that could influence the recommendations the physician makes to the patient. Finally, disclosure must specify those services not covered by the plan, including a clear definition of what is meant by "experimental or investigative treatment." Patients should be told they have the right to seek additional care outside of the plan if they are prepared to pay for it "out-of-pocket."

(e) Internal and External Appeals and Grievance Procedures. These mechanisms should be available for both subscribers and physicians to resolve disagreements and disputes about appropriate care. Most of these requirements for good practice within health care organizations are included in the various forms of patient's rights bills that state and federal legislatures have debated.

4.3.5 Organizational Ethics

Clinical care typically takes place within an organization. Care is given in hospitals or clinics, within MCOs, and within the financial constraints posed by insurers. In recent years, the concept of organizational ethics has emerged and has been encouraged by the Joint Commission for Accreditation of Health Care Organizations (JCAHO), which now requires their accredited institutions to develop programs in organizational ethics. Organizational ethics is a version of business ethics. It is the effort on the part of management and staff to express the value assumptions that should guide business or policy decisions within their institutions. Institutions should have a clear policy and programs regarding their mission, range of service, continuous quality improvement in care of patients, guidance on difficult clinical problems, and processes for dispute resolution. There should be institutional mechanisms to formulate, revise, and oversee the implementation of these policies and programs. Many of the problems noted in succeeding sections can be well-managed only within such policies and programs.

Special Issue on Organizational Ethics. *J Clin Ethics* 1999;10(3).

Special Section on Organizational Ethics in Health Care. *Camb Q Healthc Ethics* 2000;9(2).

The Patient's Bill of Rights that has been proposed for federal legislation is, in effect, an example of organizational ethics. Most proposed versions of this Bill of Rights concern such issues as access to specialists or emergency care within HMOs, appeals of coverage decisions, protection of whistle-blowers regarding HMO quality of care, and the liability of HMOs for treatment decisions that cause harm. These issues are matters for institutional policy and structure rather than problems in clinical ethics, although the discussion of physician loyalty in this chapter may provide the ethical basis for organizational ethics and for a true understanding of the rights of patients.

4.3.6 Cost Considerations in Reaching Clinical Decisions

In general: (a) Patient-centered care that focuses on medical indications and patient preferences should retain priority. This statement merely affirms the traditional responsibility of the physician to place the patient's interest before self-interest and to respect the patient's right of choice. Quality of care should not be subordinated to cost considerations but should be based on clinical data, outcome studies, and practice guidelines. Quality care does not mean, however, all available care. The clinical zeal that does everything for everybody is poor medicine. Medicine that emphasizes the methods of primary care and sound clinical judgment is often the best and most parsimonious medicine. Quality care refers to care that not only must be diagnostically sound and technically correct but that also must be appropriate. Appropriate care provides no more and no less care than is reasonably suited to the clinical problem. Such care should also be cost-effective; that is, it should be the least costly way to achieve an equal outcome. It also should be ethical; that is, it should be in accordance with ethical criteria, such as those discussed in this book.

(b) The important elements of the patient-physician relationship should be preserved. Managed care has the potential for creating conflicts of interest that divide the physician's allegiance between the patient and the health system and that place great stress on the patient-physician relationship. The physician's knowledge of the patient and the patient's trust and confidence in the physician must be preserved. This can be achieved by reinforcing the role of the physician as advocate for the patient. Health care organizations should expect physicians to argue for policies that provide all services that have a reasonable likelihood of benefiting the patient. If organizations are unable or unwilling to provide some potentially beneficial services, its physicians then have a responsibility to inform patients of these limitations and of the possibility of going outside the plan at their own cost.

(c) Patient and physician autonomy and freedom of choice should be maximized within the limits of the system. While acknowledging constraints on patient and physician preferences, ways should be devised to maximize autonomy within increasingly complex bureaucratic systems. Persons should be fully informed of the constraints of the system before choosing it. For example, if the plan does not cover "experimental treatment," patients should be given a clear definition of what is meant by "experimental treatment." Also, plans should disclose any financial incentive arrangements that exist between the plan and its physicians. To the extent possible, such incentive arrangements should be based on quality of care rather than on underutilization of care services. Physicians should be aware of the plan's quality of care, philosophy of care, and incentive structure before joining it. There should be a formal appeals process where patients' and physicians' views and grievances can be expressed and adjudicated.

(d) The system adopted by any plan should reflect principles of just distribution, ensuring that all who have a fair claim to service should receive it without discrimination. All participants in a plan, subscribers and providers, should understand and appreciate these principles. Plans would be wise to invite their members to participate in formulating a philosophy of just care.

Council of Ethical and Judicial Affairs, American Medical Association. Ethical issues in managed care. *JAMA* 1995;273:330–335.

(e) When financial incentives are available to a physician in a capitation plan, the following guidelines have been proposed to reduce the conflict of interest between clinically appropriate care and the physician's financial interest: (1) The contract should provide that less than 10% of the physician's annual income should be at risk; (2) there should be a stop-loss provision; (3) groups of physicians rather than individuals should share the risk; (4) bonuses and withholds should be calculated rarely and paid on a scale; (5) incentives should be provided for improvements in access, prevention, and patient satisfaction; and (6) risk adjustments should be made to capitation rates.

Pearson SD, Sabin JE, Emanuel EJ. Ethical guidelines for physician compensation based on capitation. *N Eng J Med* 1998;339:689–693.

Case I. Mr. S.T., a 52-year-old man with a 3-year history of diabetes and a strong family history of ischemic heart disease, complains to his primary physician at an HMO of having 3 weeks of substernal pressure that sometimes occurs at rest. The resting electrocardiogram is normal. The patient requests a referral to a cardiologist. Instead, his primary physician orders a multistage exercise test (MSET) but does not include the more sensitive and expensive thallium scintigram for evaluation of chest pain. After a borderline MSET, the patient again insists on a cardiology referral, and finally the referral is made. After completing a thallium stress test, which is borderline, the cardiologist decides to treat the patient medically instead of referring the patient to an interventional cardiologist for a coronary angiogram and possible interventions that could include angioplasty or bypass graft surgery. The HMO to which the patient, primary physician, and cardiologist belong is one that distributes a share of the annual profits to physicians if medical care expenditures are kept below a certain level.

COMMENT. The primary care physician and cardiologist face conflicts of interest. Their personal financial benefits are based partly on restricting costly services, such as thallium scans, coronary angiography, and coronary bypass graft surgery. On the other hand, their professional responsibilities to the patient require that they provide the patient with the best medical or surgical recommendations, even if these involve a costly surgical procedure. If the patient had three-vessel disease, the cardiologist would act unethically and incompetently if she did not recommend surgery. Two-vessel coronary disease and the use of thallium scans are, in contrast, both gray areas in which considerable technical disagreement remains about appropriate use, and wide variation in practice exists. In such circumstances, either decision by the HMO cardiologist would be defensible.

Ultimately, many of these dilemmas will be resolved by better outcome data. For the present, we must recognize that in gray areas, where physician practice varies, HMO physicians are likely to opt for the least costly alternative. This is ethically defensible, because persons join HMOs for the financial advantages of membership, as well as the expectation of good care. The financial solvency of such plans is a matter of common interest to all members, and hence, cost-effective care is in the interests of all. Plan members, however, should be informed that the plan encourages cost-effective care within the context of appropriate care. They should also be told that they can go outside the plan, at their own cost, to seek forms of care that are not recommended or provided within the plan. Public opinion is reacting against some of the more egregious practices of MCOs, such as restrictive referrals and denying or limiting hospital stays. Medicare and Medicaid regulations and states' laws prohibit certain other practices, such as direct payment incentives for limiting care. Still, even as organizational practices and policies are made more conformable with the demands of ethics and quality, certain ethical problems will remain.

4.4 ALLOCATION OF SCARCE HEALTH RESOURCES

Allocation of scarce resources is sometimes called "rationing." Rationing can have the broad meaning of distributing any limited resource by any allocation mechanism, such as the market. It may have the more specific meaning of allocating some limited resource by a plan stating criteria and priorities. Gasoline and food rationing in wartime are rationing of this more specific type. Health care in the United States has long been rationed by the market, and in accord with implicit rather than explicit criteria. The number of physicians, the location of their practices, the ability of persons to pay, and the different perceptions of medical need—these factors and many others result in medical resources being allocated in certain ways that can result in certain allocations and constitute implicit rationing. In recent years, the question has been raised whether medical resources should be allocated by explicit criteria. For example, the state of Oregon established priorities according to which particular treatments for particular disease conditions would be reimbursed by Medicaid. This question belongs to the ethics of health policy and is not discussed in this book. However, any such policy will have effects at the clinical level. Whether physicians should make allocation decisions by balancing societal efficiency against the interests of individual patients will then become a topic for consideration.

Beauchamp TL, Childress JF. Justice. In: *Principles of Biomedical Ethics.* 5th ed. New York: Oxford University Press; 2001:225–272.

Kilner JF. *Who Lives? Who Dies? Ethical Criteria in Patient Selection.* New Haven: Yale University Press; 1990.

Case. Mr. D.P., a 75-year-old man with a long history of heart disease and diabetes, is admitted to an ICU with fever, hypotension, and shortness of breath. The chest film is consistent with ARDS, and the Po_2 is 50 mm Hg. At morning rounds, the intern asks whether this aggressive, costly treatment is appropriate for an elderly man who has underlying heart disease and diabetes and whose chances of recovering unimpaired from this episode may be no greater than 35%. At noon conference, the attending physician asks the house officers whether they should provide indicated treatment or should they begin rationing health care by making tough choices, starting immediately with this elderly man?

COMMENT. The easiest form of rationing for individual physicians—and the least problematic ethically—involves forgoing medical activities that are useless or unnecessary. Costly, scarce resources should not be expended wastefully on patients who will not benefit. Of course, determining when a particular form of intervention is likely to be use-less, unnecessary, or only marginally beneficial requires acute clinical judgment and is often impossible. The recent trend toward outcome studies and clinical epidemiology can be helpful. The clinician must base clinical judgments on medical indications and patient preferences, and less on quality-of-life factors, such as age, mental status, or financial resources. The problem, as illustrated in the case of the 75-year-old man (who subsequently recovered without any impairment), is that at the time of his admission to the hospital, physicians could not be certain whether they were dealing with someone who was "terminally ill" or whether they were dealing with someone, as the case turned out, who was critically ill but had prospects of recovering completely.

4.4.1 Admission to Programs with Limited Resources

The entire health care system strains under ever-increasing needs and de-mands for service. Certain procedures and therapeutic programs are available only at a few locales or from a few specialists. More persons may need a certain sort of care than can be accommodated. Certain resources, such as funds for unreimbursed care, physician's time, availability of op-erating rooms, and the like, are relatively scarce; that is, society can make choices that would increase the availability of these resources. Other re-sources, such as life saving solid organs, such as livers or hearts, are ab-solutely scarce; that is, even with good social policy about their acquisi-tion and distribution, there will always be fewer than needed. How should health care resources be allocated? Although this is a policy ques-tion that this book generally avoids, the allocation of scarce resources is one policy that directly affects patient care. All commentators on the ethics of this problem agree that resources should be allocated in a fair manner. What constitutes fairness? One of the landmark events in recent medical history offers an example.

EXAMPLE. When chronic hemodialysis became available in the 1960s, the limited resources required some rationing device. A local committee was established to screen all applicants who had been judged acceptable on medical grounds. The committee relied on "social worth" criteria, that is, personal and social characteristics that merited the treatment. This tech-nique proved unworkable and was much criticized for bias and prejudice.

COMMENT. Extensive ethical discussion of this issue seems to have reached consensus on the unacceptability of social worth as a principle of fair distribution. The danger of bias and prejudice in a social worth system advises its rejection as a rationing device. Some commentators have favored "queuing" (first come, first served), although they note that these systems favor the better informed and better connected, who can hurry to the queue. Many favor a lottery, whereby all participate in a drawing of random numbers. This system, however, is faulted, because the pool of needy persons does not exist at any one time.

It seems fair to establish certain basic objective criteria—for example, medical condition, potential for benefit, and age—and within a pool of those who meet these criteria to select randomly. It may also be useful to establish a "due process" system that could make exceptions to these criteria.

4.4.2 Triage

Medical care has long been provided in accordance with a rationing plan in one specific situation, battlefield medicine. In recent years, triage rules have been refined and applied to other disasters, such as earthquakes and hurricanes. The rules of triage and its rationale are stated in a hand-book of military surgery as follows:

> Priority is to be given to (1) slightly injured who can be quickly re-turned to service, (2) the more seriously injured who demand imme-diate resuscitation or surgery, (3) the "hopelessly wounded. . . . The military surgeon must expend his energies in the treatment of only those whose survival seems likely, in line with the objective of mili-tary medicine, which has been defined as "doing the greatest good for the greatest number" in the proper time and place.

> *Emergency War Surgery.* Washington, DC: Government Printing Office, 1958.

COMMENT. The ethical basis for military triage is to return to service those who are needed for victory, a common good for the army and the nation. Similarly, disaster triage provides priority to persons such as fire-fighters, public safety officers, and medical personnel in order for them to be returned to rescue work. Present disaster and serious danger to the society justify triage rules. Lacking the element of present disaster and the destruction of the fabric of social order, rules that subordinate the needs of individuals to the needs of society are not easily justified in medical ethics.

4.4.3 Allocation of Solid Organs for Transplantation

Organ transplantation is one of the greatest achievements of modern medicine. For the first time in history, individuals with failure of vital or-gans such as heart, kidney, and liver can be saved from certain death by the timely transplantation of a donated organ. The essential ethical prin-ciple of organ transplant requires that the organ be a true "donation," that is, a gift voluntarily and altruistically given by the donor to the recipient. A living donor may make this gift, as is often done between relatives in kidney transplantation and, increasingly, in liver transplantation, or a person may designate that their organs be used after their death, a practice approved by American law. The Uniform Anatomical Gift Act, adopted by all states, provides a system for identification of donors (usually noted on driver's licenses). Organs cannot be "harvested" from the dead without prior authorization of the deceased or, after death, by next of kin. Most transplanted organs are obtained from persons declared dead by brain criteria, but in recent years, because the number of cadaveric donors has remained constant and inadequate, an increasing number of organs are obtained from related or unrelated living donors or from an expanded cadaveric donor pool that includes marginal donors and non–heart-beating donors. Many state laws require physicians to request organ donation from the family of the newly deceased (an emotionally difficult but necessary task).

Despite these efforts to increase organ donation, the demand for solid organs far exceeds supply. In the United States in 2000, 23,000 organ transplants were performed. At the end of 2001, 78,000 persons were on the waiting lists for all organs. Six thousand people died while on the waiting list. Thus, a fair and equitable distribution system must be created and maintained. The key elements of such a system are (1) it avoids social worth criteria; (2) it recognizes the patient's potential for benefit; (3) it has a place for urgency of need; (4) it avoids discrimination based on sex, race, or social status; and (5) it employs a transparent process perceived by the public as fair.

In the United States, a government-supported private organization, the United Network on Organ Sharing (UNOS), manages the distribution of organs. UNOS policy allocates organs on the basis of medical status, blood type, time on the waiting list, and geographic distance between donor and recipient. A computerized system manages these data. Its policies about organ retrieval and distribution can be obtained on line.

UNOS: http://www.unos.org.

Special Issue on Organ Transplantation: Shaping Policy and Keeping Public Trust. *Camb Q Healthc Ethics* 1999;8(3).

Special Section on Organ Transplantation. *Hastings Cent Rep* 1999;29(6).

Case I. J.J. is a 50-year-old man with end-stage liver disease caused by primary biliary cirrhosis. He has experienced several complications in recent years, including portal hypertension, bleeding gastric varices, ascites, and one episode of encephalopathy. He has been on the liver transplant waiting list for 3 years, but because the geographic region in which he lives has long waiting times and because he has blood type O, it may be 2 years before a matched organ becomes available. Because livers are allocated partly by medical urgency, and because J.J.'s physician is concerned that he may die of complications of liver failure, the physician proposes to increase the chance of getting a liver by admitting him to the ICU, which gives him a higher priority. This means that J.J. jumps the queue and may qualify for a liver within a week. The admission to the ICU is accomplished by diagnosing a grade 3 encephalopathy, which is quickly reversed by treatment, and then keeping him in the unit until the liver becomes available. Some describe this as "gaming the system."

COMMENT. Is it ethical for the physician to "game the system" to improve the patient's chance for a life saving transplantation? The physician argues that J.J.'s region and blood type place him at a disadvantage. "Gaming" simply gives him the same chance as someone who lives in a region with shorter lists and with a more common blood type. We disagree with this behavior and its rationale. Although physicians have a duty to advocate for their patients, the limits of that advocacy are honestly devised arrangements for a just and fair distribution of social benefits. The leveling of the playing field should be done by policy, not by clinical decisions. Since the late 1990, UNOS and the Federal government have been debating ways to even out the obvious disparities between regional waiting times and to balance long waits with urgency. Also, gaming is usually a skill of the socially and economically competent, introducing serious discrimination into a system meant to overcome it. Thus, despite the hardships and even threat of death, J.J. and his physician should play by the rules.

Case II. J.J. has been waiting for 2 years for a liver transplant. He visits his surgeon's office with a person whom he introduces as "my best friend" and says he has read about some transplant programs that use living donors for segmental liver transplants. J.J.'s friend says that he would like to volunteer as a living donor. The surgeon has several concerns: (1) Should a healthy person be subjected to the substantial risks of morbidity and mortality associated with transplant surgery? (2) Because the surgeon has not performed a living donor procedure, should J.J. be referred to one of the US programs that has a record of such procedures? (3) Can the surgeon verify that this person is really a "best friend" or a hired "volunteer" who has agreed to donate for a fee? and (4) Should the surgeon do the detective work to determine the truth of the matter?

COMMENT. Although living persons have been kidney donors since the earliest days of transplantation, ethical questions remain about the ethics of surgery on a healthy person to benefit another. This practice has been deemed ethical if the donor is an informed, free, and uncoerced volunteer, aware of the risks involved in this operation. Segmental liver transplant involves a higher risk than kidney transplantation. Also, obtaining organs by purchase is illegal in the United States. Thus, it must be very clear that Mr. J.J.'s friend is an informed, free, and uncoerced donor. The surgeon should converse privately with the volunteer, informing him of the risks of the surgery. A physician not related to the case should be asked to be a "donor advocate" to explore more deeply the possibility of coercion and medical suitability. Any suspicion of coercion or of financial incentive disqualifies the volunteer. Also, the surgeon should refer the case to a program with more experience in living donor operations.

4.4.3 P Organ Transplantation for Children

Successful organ transplantation depends on having donors that are HLA-compatible. Such donors are often siblings. Thus, one may ask, "Is it ethical to take a kidney or bone marrow from a healthy child for a seriously ill sibling?" In the first recorded case, this question had an inauspicious answer, because the healthy donor was a retarded child, thus creating suspicion that the retarded are to be devalued and used for the benefit of others. The major question, however, is the risk to which a healthy child is put for the possible benefit of another. In our view, it is indefensible to impose the serious risk of removal of a kidney; it is defensible to suggest the notably less serious risks of donation of bone marrow. Needless to say, the negotiations with family and with the child require the utmost delicacy, the psychologic implications for the children in the event of either failure or success must be recognized, and the legal requirements in the jurisdiction must be complied with. Should there be parental disagreement, the plan should be abandoned.

4.4.4 Competing Claims to Care

Situations can occur where it can be asked whether the claims of one patient for care override the claims of another. Personnel, time, equipment, beds, and other factors may be insufficient to accommodate both. In addition, the fundamental ethical justification for triage, namely, contribution to social good, is not present; this is a competition between two rival claimants.

Case I. Mrs. C.Z. is a 71-year-old woman who has a diagnosed lung tumor for which she refused surgery. She developed obstructive pneumonia and was admitted to the ICU of the community hospital in her rural county. She has shown no signs of improvement for 7 days. She is now obtunded. The victim of an automobile accident is brought to the hospital with a crushed chest, apparent pneumothorax, and broken bones in the extremities. This trauma patient requires a respirator immediately. Mrs. C.Z., of the six patients on the six respirators in the ICU, has the poorest prognosis. She seems unable to be weaned and thus would probably die if ventilatory support were discontinued. Should she be removed in favor of the accident victim?

COMMENT. The medical prognosis of Mrs. C.Z. is poor. She has cancer of the lung with bronchial obstruction and pneumonia that has failed to respond to treatment. She is comatose and likely to die within days. She is now incapable of expressing preferences. Nothing is known about her preferences, except her refusal of surgery. Given these considerations, the immediate and serious need of an identifiable other person becomes an important consideration. When that person also is in imminent danger of death, the contextual factor of scarcity of resources becomes decisive in the decision regarding Mrs. C.Z. In theory, it is ethically permissible to recommend that respiratory support be discontinued. In practice, when the resources are only relatively scarce, these situations usually are managed on the scene, by such practices as calling in additional ICU nurses or by making exceptions to the rule about use of ventilators outside the ICU. Such practical stratagems often resolve ethical problems.

Case II. Patient R.A., the drug addict described at Section 2.9.2, is in need of a second prosthetic heart valve. Several physicians are strongly opposed to providing a second prosthesis. These physicians offer three reasons: (1) Surgery is futile, because the patient will become reinfected; (2) the patient does not care enough about himself to follow a regimen or to abstain from drugs; and (3) it is a poor use of societal resources.

COMMENT. The first and second considerations are discussed in Sections 1.1.3 and 2.9. The third consideration raises the following new ethical issues:

(a) What are the criteria for differentiating good from poor uses of societal resources? Although such criteria might be formulated at the policy level, it is impossible to do so at the clinical level because the overall view of social need and the contribution of particular decisions to that need are not known to clinicians. Also, attempts to formulate such criteria risk introducing serious bias and discrimination into clinical decisions.

(b) There is no guarantee that whatever is "saved" by refusing this patient will be used in any better manner. The societal resources are, of course, not being "absorbed" only by the patient. Instead, they are flowing to the hospital, to the physicians and surgeons, to nurses, and so on.

RECOMMENDATION. The most acceptable ethical justification for refusing to provide a second prosthesis is the medical indication that the risk of surgery with its attendant mortality rate exceeds the risk of managing the patient with medical therapy. Thus, if medically indicated, the surgery should be offered. The ethical obligation to provide surgical assistance is, however, diminished to the extent that the rights of other patients are directly compromised, as explained in the comment to Case I.

4.5 RELIGION

Religious belief and the teachings of various faith communities are relevant to medical care. Religion offers powerful perspectives on suffering, loss, and death. The majority of Americans profess some form of religious belief. Also, many persons from other cultures are deeply committed to their religious traditions. Experience reveals the value of religious belief in times of sickness and death. Religious counselors and chaplains have an important role to play in health care. However, Western medicine has long maintained a distance from religion because of scientific skepticism about faith and the professional duty to avoid favoritism toward any religious position. Nevertheless, many physicians respect the tenets of their own religion and allow them to influence their practice of medicine. Catholicism and Judaism both have extensive teachings about health and medical care that may dictate or prohibit certain interventions. However, today persons holding many forms of religious and spiritual beliefs, often unfamiliar to providers, appear in American health care settings. Thus, the place of religion in clinical ethics is complex. We have already noted the problems raised for clinical ethics when patients adhere to beliefs that repudiate medical treatment (Chapter 2). Here we note some other aspects of religion in clinical care.

Case I. Mr. M.R., a 66-year-old man, has just had a Whipple procedure for pancreatic cancer. His recovery from the surgery has been difficult, and 2 weeks after surgery, he remains in the hospital. His family, Mrs. R., and five adult children, are faithfully present in his hospital room. They are all devout Christians. Dr. K., the surgeon, makes rounds twice daily. Each time he comes into the room, the family ask him to pray with them for Mr. R's recovery. Dr. K. has no religious affiliation. On one visit, one of Mr. R's sons shows Dr. K. an article he has found from the medical literature, claiming that research has shown that patients for whom regular prayer is offered recover more quickly. He reiterates the family's invitation to common prayer.

Case II. Dr. N.A. is a family practitioner, who also is board certified in obstetrics and gynecology. She is on the staff of a clinic in a neighborhood that has a large population of Ethiopian and Somalian immigrants. Dr. N.A. has earned the trust of women in that community because of her sympathetic understanding of their way of life. She herself was brought up as a Black Muslim and has studied the Koran and classical Islamic tradition. A delegation of Somalian women visit her and ask whether she will regularly perform ritual genital surgery on the young women of the community. That surgery, commonly called clitoridectomy, and referred to by its opponents as genital mutilation, is now done by medically untrained women. Her visitors suppose that she understands that this ritual is required for any devout Muslim woman. Dr. N.A. has seen the medical problems consequent on this procedure. She is repelled by it and knows from her own study of Islamic law that it is not required by the Koran or by the traditions of the prophet.

RECOMMENDATION. In Case I, the surgeon should show respect for the family's spiritual beliefs and politely decline to pray with them, saying something like, "I do know about the study you mention, but I doubt that the prayers of an unbeliever would be helpful." He might tell them that he will convey their wishes to his colleague physicians and hospital chaplains. If any physician feels comfortable joining the family in prayer, it is appropriate to do so. The primary issue is to avoid depreciation of spiritual beliefs that cannot harm and may help.

In Case II, Dr. N.A. is faced with a moral dilemma. She does not wish to lose the confidence of women who badly need a sympathetic physician. She does not want to see young women mutilated by crudely performed procedures. She does not want to be complicit in a ritual that serves male domination. Still, her own moral repugnance, coupled with the fact that this surgery does not meet professional standards, should incline her to refuse, attempting at the same time to educate these women both about the religious law of their own faith and the medical consequences of the practice.

4.6   THE ROLE OF THE LAW IN CLINICAL ETHICS

The law has been mentioned many times in this book on ethics. The practice of medicine has long been the subject of legislation, and many judicial cases have involved medical practice, particularly when physicians are accused of negligence. In recent years, the volume of legislation, litigation, and regulation around medicine and health care has increased notably. Health care providers should be educated about the ways in which law and ethics intersect and overlap in medical practice. Although health professionals rarely have technical or detailed knowledge of the law, they should be able to identify potential legal issues and know when to seek legal guidance. For example, topics such as informed consent, confidentiality, advance directives, and many other issues discussed in this book have both ethical and legal aspects.

When ethical conflicts occur in health care, legal rules may sometimes set limits to ethical options or even create ethical conflicts. For instance, laws may prohibit assisted suicide by making it a crime for physicians to provide the means, such as a lethal dose of barbiturates, for patients to take their own lives. In Oregon, however, physicians are permitted by state law to prescribe barbiturates for competent, terminally ill patients who meet eligibility and procedural requirements. Similarly, a few statutes permit physicians to prescribe "medical marijuana" for AIDS and cancer patients, but the United States Attorney General has successfully challenged these statutes as violations of federal controlled substances laws. Health professionals may sometimes feel conflicted between the ethical duty to protect confidential communication and legal duties to make required reports to protect public health or safety. In general, codes of professional ethics impose upon professionals the duty to obey the law. Occasionally, a physician may make a conscientious judgment that the law impedes a strong ethical duty. If the physician acts in accord with this judgment, he or she is a conscientious objector and should accept the legal consequences.

Physicians may sometimes feel frustrated by laws that seem burdensome, such as reporting requirements or limitations on access to care. In specific cases, physicians may seek authorization for making an exception to usual legal requirements or seek clarification of their precise legal obligations. Physicians occasionally falsely believe or assert that the law imposes duties that are not required. Also, some physicians have an inordinate and uninformed fear of liability. Studies have shown that physicians may seek legal information from highly unreliable sources, namely, from other physicians.

McCreary SV, Swanson JW, Perkins HS, et al. Treatment decisions for terminally ill patients: Physicians' legal defensiveness and knowledge of medical law. *Law Med Health Care* 1992;20:364–376.

When questions arise about legal regulation of medical practice, it is prudent to seek expert advice. When questions arise about potential conflicts between ethical values and legal obligations, physicians should use institutional means, such as ethics consultation, committees, legal services, or professional organizations, to clarify their options and responsibilities.

A common fault is to allow a discussion of the law to preempt an ethical discussion. Although legal issues may be relevant to the case, they do not settle an ethical problem that must be discussed in the framework for ethical analysis proposed in this book.

4.6 P Law and Pediatrics

Certain laws particularly affect the care of infants and children. All states have passed child protection legislation that requires providers to report to authorities instances of suspected abuse and neglect of children. Two federal laws, one statutory and the other judicial, also pertain to clinical decisions made by pediatricians. In 1985, the US Congress passed amendments to The Child Abuse Prevention and Treatment and Adoption Reform Act. These amendments, commonly known as the "Baby Doe Rules," set certain legal standards for clinical decisions regarding the care of the newborn infant. We have mentioned these rules under the topics where they apply (Sections 1.4 P, 2.7.3 P, 3.0.1 P, and 3.2 P). The Baby Doe Rules are not addressed directly to providers of neonatal care; they apply to state Child Protective Agencies, which are required to monitor their observance by hospitals. Neonatologists are advised to seek interpretation of these rules from local legal counsel.

A recent controversial court decision about medical care for an anencephalic infant was based on federal legislation designed to guarantee appropriate emergency care for indigent patients. Baby K. was born anencephalic. Her mother, who had strong, religiously based vitalistic beliefs, chose to take her home for the remainder of her expected short life. When the baby experienced, as would be expected, serious respiratory distress, the mother brought her to the hospital emergency department for treatment. Although reluctant to provide treatment that the physicians judged futile, the hospital did so, but then petitioned the court for relief. The court found that the federal Emergency Medical Treatment and Active Labor Act (EMTALA), a federal law requiring hospitals to stabilize emergency patients before transferring them, obliged the hospital to provide medical care for Baby K. In this case, the mother's beliefs and hopes prevailed over the hospital's claim that continued ventilator support was futile. It is difficult to generalize from this peculiar case to the broad problem of defining the futility of treatment (see Section 1.1.3). Finally, as mentioned at Section 2.5.1 P, many states have enacted provisions that permit an exemption to the usual child and neglect charges or to specific provisions, such as required school immunization.

4.7 CLINICAL RESEARCH

Clinical research is essential to modern medicine; new therapeutic and diagnostic interventions must be tested and evaluated by applying them to humans, and often those humans must be patients, persons suffering from the disease for which the intervention is designed. In the past, patients were often unwilling and unknowing subjects of clinical research.

Today, this is ethically and legally unacceptable, and research is clearly distinguished from treatment. Physicians must know how that distinction is made and be aware of their responsibilities when they undertake clinical research.

Beauchamp TL, Childress JF. The dual roles of physician and investigator. In: *Principles of Biomedical Ethics.* 5th ed. New York: Oxford University Press; 2001:319–328.

Levine RJ. *Ethics and Regulation of Clinical Research.* New Haven: Yale University Press; 1986.

IRB: *Ethics and Human Research.* The Hastings Center, Garrison, New York.

4.7.1 Definition of Clinical Research

Clinical research is defined as any clinical intervention involving human subjects, patients or normal volunteers, performed in accordance with a protocol designed to yield generalizable scientific knowledge. The protocol sets out the research techniques, such as randomization and double blinding, and the statistical techniques necessary to establish validity of the data. The benefits of research accrue to persons other than the subject of research, namely, to future patients, to the professional doing the research, and to society in general. Even when the subject personally benefits—for example, a cancer goes into remission as the possible result of treatment with an experimental drug—these others benefit from the knowledge produced by the research. The research protocol is usually designed as a clinical trial, in which patients are randomized to the investigative intervention or to an alternative, such as a placebo or to current best treatment. This randomization is ethically justified by "clinical equipoise," that is, the opinion of the relevant community of experts that, on the basis of available evidence, there is no difference between the trial intervention and alternatives. The purpose of the research is to demonstrate that this assumption is correct or is wrong in favor of one or the other treatment. In addition, patients and usually investigators are not aware of which intervention the research subject is receiving.

4.7.2 Regulation of Clinical Research

Clinical research is governed by guidelines promulgated in several ethical statements, principally the Nuremberg Code, the Helsinki Declaration of the World Medical Association, and the Belmont Report. Regulations promulgated by the US Department of Health and Human Services are mandatory for all research done in institutions that receive federal funds and also for research done in private industry that will be submitted for FDA approval.

45 *Code Of Federal Regulations* 46:1981; 48:1983.

Sugarman J, Mastroianni AC, Kahn JP (eds). *Ethics of Research with Human Subjects. Selected Policies and Resources.* Frederick, Md: University Publishing Co; 1998.

The following actions are required by these regulations:

(a) Review of proposed research by an institutional review board (IRB). The IRB consists of persons competent to understand the science of the protocol and other informed persons, some of whom should be independent of the institution. This IRB must evaluate the protocol design, assess the risks and benefits of the research procedures, and recommend approval or disapproval to the funding agency. Many of the ethical problems regarding research must be resolved in the course of the review, for example, an appropriate risk/benefit ratio, the details of informed consent, and the suitability of compensation.

(b) Informed consent by any competent participant or permission by surrogates for incapacitated persons without decision-making capability (with special review and protection procedures for specific cases). Consent must stress the voluntary nature of participation in research and indicate that the patient's refusal will not compromise the care and attention due to all patients. Coercion, caused by excessive compensation or to the professional authority of the researcher, must be avoided.

(c) Fair selection of subjects. Attention must be paid to the selection of appropriate populations as research subjects; that is, researchers must avoid taking advantage of vulnerable populations and must achieve racial and gender balance, to the extent compatible with the objectives of the protocol.

4.7.3 Innovative Treatment

Most clinical activity involves familiar procedures and medications; relatively few of these have undergone the close scrutiny of a formally designed clinical trial. Their efficacy is attested only by cumulative experience. New treatments are constantly being devised by commercial firms and by individual physicians.

EXAMPLE. Physicians may choose to use a drug that has FDA approval for one indication for another condition in which it has never been used ("off-label use"). Surgeons may modify a standard surgical maneuver or create an entirely new one.

COMMENT. Clinicians may use such methods in the care of a particular patient. They should do so prudently, with solid conviction that the new use or procedure is likely to be safe and effective. This is called "innovative treatment." It is not research, because the use is not designed to produce generalizable information, even though a clinician might be able to draw conclusions in retrospect. Innovative treatment is not, as such, governed by the codes and regulations that govern research. However, it should be governed by the same spirit. The advice of knowledgeable colleagues should be sought, a risk/benefit ratio as accurate as possible should be worked out, and the consent of the patient to be the recipient of yet untried treatment should be obtained. In addition, innovative treatment should be designed as closely as possible to research, so that the social benefit of valid knowledge can be obtained. Finally, in doubtful cases, clinicians should seek the advice of the IRB about the advisability of innovative treatment. Misjudgment in using innovative treatment can lead to malpractice charges.

"Investigational treatment" describes forms of diagnosis and therapy that are under development and have not reached the stage where a formally designed clinical trial can demonstrate efficacy. Development is fostered because existing data suggest that the treatment is "promising." Patients suffering from a condition for which no effective therapy exists may seek such promising treatment, and their physicians, even if skeptical about its efficacy, may be eager to offer hope. Third-party payers usually explicitly exclude investigational (sometimes called "experimental") treatment from coverage and managed care organizations discourage its use. However, some insurers and health care organizations are willing to consider payment for investigational treatments that are promising, on a showing of clinical appropriateness.

EXAMPLE. Hematopoietic stem cell transplantation is rapidly developing as a therapy for many malignancies. Autologous stem cell transplantation has been proven curative for relapsed Hodgkin's and non-Hodgkin's lymphoma, relapsed and high-risk initial acute myelogenous and lymphocytic leukemia, and multiple myeloma; remission has been effected in other conditions, such as chronic myelogenous leukemia and aplastic anemia. However, it is still in the early experimental stage for many other conditions, such as primary amyloidosis. Allogeneic transplant, necessary when the patient cannot provide his or her own bone marrow, has much less efficacy for any condition. Still, many patients and their doctors consider these investigative procedures as a last hope in refractory disease. Even the high risk of death associated with bone marrow ablation does not deter them, because patients face death from their disease.

COMMENT. Investigational treatments should be recommended with great caution. Their promise is often unfulfilled, and their negative effects are sometimes hidden. At the same time, patients may have no other recourse, and medicine advances by these tentative steps.

Physicians should make every effort to ensure that their patients see these treatments in a realistic light. Administrators of health plans should make clear the policy of their organization relative to provision and reimbursement and establish means of assessing treatment. In the 1990s, reports of favorable results from high-dose chemotherapy followed by stem cell transplant for advanced breast cancer prompted many women and their doctors to seek this highly investigative and highly risky procedure. Pressure from patients and from judicial decisions forced insurers to cover the procedure. When investigative studies were completed, it became clear that the procedure offered no advantage over standard treatment and had much higher adverse effects. Thus, the hope of many patients for cure or remission ended not only with disappointment, but their death may also have been hastened by the procedure.

4.7.4 Compassionate Use

While a drug is being studied in an approved research protocol, a physician may determine that, even though data do not yet confirm its efficacy and safety, it may be the only available treatment for the patient with an immediately life-threatening disease. The FDA has a provision to allow the physician and the sponsor of the new drug to petition for its use in treatment. This is commonly called "compassionate use" (although the FDA does not use this term). The physician must demonstrate a reasonable basis for believing that the drug may be effective, that its use would not expose the patient to significant additional risks, and that there is no satisfactory alternative drug. The sponsoring company must affirm that it is actively pursuing marketing approval of the drug.

4.7.5 Ethical Problems in Clinical Research

All clinician-researchers should honor the ethics of clinical research by abiding by the requirements of informed consent of subjects and review of protocols by competent bodies. However, in clinical situations ethical problems may still arise. It might be asked whether a particular patient, who is in general an appropriate candidate for an approved protocol, should be approached because the risk/benefit ratio is questionable in this patient's case. This problem might arise in situations in which a new drug, believed to be of potential benefit from preliminary animal and human investigations, is compared in a formal clinical trial with a placebo. In double-blind trials, neither the doctor nor the patient knows whether the patient is receiving a drug or placebo. Some physicians find this situation clinically and ethically unacceptable. Some physicians are concerned that their patients may be randomized to an inferior therapy. It can be asked whether patients should be continued on protocol, or new patients entered, when a clinician-researcher believes the majority of patients whom he has treated seem to benefit from one experimental drug rather than the standard treatment.

EXAMPLE I. A clinician is entering patients in a randomized double-blind trial of a drug to prevent angina. He suspects from the side effects which drug is the standard one and which is the experimental. He also has the impression that patients are doing much better on the suspected research drug than on the standard one.

COMMENT. The investigator seems caught between two obligations: the duty to benefit the patient and the contractual duty to carry out the trial (and the more abstract duty to advance medical science). In principle, the duty to benefit the patient supersedes all others. However, in this situation, suspicion and clinical impression do not override the scientifically founded uncertainty until properly collected data are analyzed. Only if the individual clinical investigator is convinced that the use or nonuse of a certain drug may cause harm does it become unethical to proceed. Soundly designed clinical trials should have oversight mechanisms (data safety monitoring boards) to monitor trends, to deal with the problems of clinical impressions, and to terminate the trial should the evidence of distinct benefit or harm become pervasive.

EXAMPLE II. A new drug is being tested to determine its efficacy in treatment of cytomegalovirus (CMV) retinitis, a frequent infection of persons with AIDS and one that can result in blindness. A strictly controlled trial has been designed to gather the most valid data possible, because the known adverse effects of the drug must be balanced by demonstrated benefits. One aspect of the control is a random allocation of patients into two groups, one of which will receive the new drug and the other a combination of the two best of the currently used drugs. A physician involved in the trial finds that certain of her patients specifically request the new drug on the grounds that AIDS advocacy literature indicates that it is more effective in preventing blindness. She wonders whether she should provide the drug outside of the controlled trial.

RECOMMENDATION. This is not an instance of compassionate use, because other treatments are available (Section 4.7.4). The investigator should not provide the drug outside the trial. The trial is based on the hypothesis that the new drug and the old drugs are equivalent; the outcome of the trial will demonstrate the superiority of one over the other, on the basis of clinical efficacy and drug toxicity. The investigator should disabuse those who seek the experimental drug of the idea that it will give them a better chance. Use of the drug outside the trial will confound the evidence necessary to demonstrate the effectiveness of the new drug.

Case III. The investigator of the cytomegalovirus drug trial is a paid consultant of the sponsoring pharmaceutical company and holds several hundred shares of the stock.

COMMENT. Conflict of interest on the part of researchers has become a focus of attention. A researcher with financial interests at stake has an incentive to modify the results of the trial, either by falsifying data or by interpreting ambiguous data to favor the trial drug. It is strongly advised, and now required by most research institutions, that investigators take the following actions: (1) disclose their financial interests to the institution and even to the research subject; (2) identify their financial affiliations in any published papers; (3) divest themselves of substantial interests; and (4) participate in mechanisms to ensure the validity of data, such as outside peer review. Physicians who have deep involvement with drug sponsors should recuse themselves as investigators for the products of that company.

4.7 P Pediatric Research

The involvement of children as research subjects was carefully studied by the National Commission for the Protection of Subjects of Biomedical and Behavioral Research. The conclusions of that commission are now embodied in federal regulations that reflect sound ethical judgments. In addition to the ethical considerations about research in general, stated in Section 4.7, pediatric research should be based on the following ethical principles:

(a) There must be sound reasons why the research must be done with children. In general, this will be because the condition under study affects only children, and no animal models suffice to study it. The results should be important for the health of children.

(b) Studies should be done in adults before children, if feasible.

(c) The level of risk to the child must be carefully assessed. If the physical and psychologic risks of research are nonexistent or minimal, that is, not exceeding the risks allowed children in daily life or the risks of routine medical exams, the research need not be justified by prospect of benefit to the child. If the risks are more than minimal, some prospect of personal benefit must be present; that is, the research must also have some therapeutic potential for the subject.

(d) Any research proposal that involves more than minimal risks and offers no personal benefit to the subject requires special review to adjudicate its vital importance for the health of children. Institutional review boards, which must approve of all research, can advise researchers about details of the requirements for ethical research involving children.

(e) The informed consent of parents or guardians, and their close involvement in the research, must be obtained. The consent of the child should also be sought when the child is at that stage of maturity where the nature of the procedure and the concept of an invitation to help others voluntarily can be understood. A child's dissent should be respected, unless the research procedure is directly associated with a necessary therapy that cannot be provided outside of research modalities.

Department of Health and Human Services Rules and Regulations. 45 *Code of Federal Regulations* 46, subpart D:1983.

Case. Amy, the girl with acute myelogenous leukemia (Section 1.2 P), received a bone marrow transplantation, after which she relapsed. Amy is a candidate for a clinical research protocol of a new drug combination. She is now aged 11 years. Her parents are eager to enter into the trial. She repeatedly and tearfully refuses.

COMMENT. Therapy and research are significantly different. Therapy promises sound hope of achieving the goal of intervention; research may offer some hope of doing so, but also has as its goal the benefit of other and future patients. A refusal of research by a child, even though it might be thought that the child, if older, would accept, should generally be honored. The National Commission for the Protection of Human Subjects of Biomedical and Behavioral Research recommended that the age of 7 years be considered as the point at which a child's consent for a research intervention be sought and refusal honored. This has been criticized as unrealistic, but it emphasizes the point that children have the right to refuse interventions that hold more promise for others than for themselves.

Most drugs used in children have been tested in adults only. Current FDA policies require pediatric drugs to be tested in children for safety and efficacy to ensure proper labeling. Generally, the effects of drugs that are used in a substantial number of children or that could be more therapeutically beneficial to children than existing therapies, and could pose a significant risk to the children if inadequately labeled, must be studied in children. Researchers are encouraged to study the effects of investigational compounds in children to determine proper dosing. Because drug companies are granted extensions of patent for testing drugs in children, large trials are now being mounted. Pediatricians in practice are solicited to conduct these trials with their patients. When any practitioner is approached, he or she should be certain that the proper IRB review has been done and that the assessment of risk and benefit is clearly delineated. They should ask for copies of the IRB review before accepting a contract. The Academy of Pediatrics has produced guidelines for practitioners acting as investigators.

Guidelines for the ethical conduct of studies to evaluate drugs in pediatric populations. Committee on Drugs, American Academy of Pediatrics. *Pediatrics* 1995;95:286–294.

4.8 CLINICAL TEACHING

Many patients receive care in institutions where clinical teaching is done. Their disease and its diagnosis and treatment provide an opportunity for students in the health sciences to learn the skills necessary for their profession. Often, treatment will be provided by a student. It is possible that some clinical decisions are made with a view to teaching and that such decisions may conflict with the patient's interests and/or wishes.

4.8.1 Consent to Be a Teaching Subject

Persons who enter teaching hospitals usually sign a general consent to that effect. Many patients, particularly those who are seriously ill at the time of admission, or who, for other reasons, cannot comprehend the meaning of the teaching hospital consent form, have probably not given adequate informed consent to be used as teaching subjects. They should be asked specifically about each episode of teaching and invited to participate. The fact that a particular procedure will be done by a student, and that it is for teaching rather than for their care or in addition to their care, should be made clear. The request should be made politely and a refusal accepted graciously. Patients are amazingly generous in consenting to participate in the education of medical students in teaching hospitals.

On occasion of the medical school course on history taking and physical diagnosis, many patients provide their histories to five or more students and allow their bodies to be prodded without complaint. In the light of these observations, it is particularly important that, when the occasional patient refuses to participate in one or another teaching exercise, the student and the faculty respect the patient's wishes absolutely and not threaten or intimidate the patient in any way. Medical students and physicians must remember that individual patients are not obligated to participate in the training of society's future physicians. They almost invariably are eager to do so. Clinical teachers and students should be grateful of patients' unquestioning generosity.

Case I. A 52-year-old obese woman required a lumbar puncture. She had, on admission, signed a general consent to teaching procedures that did not specify who would perform them. A second-year resident entered her room with two medical students. He told the patient that she needed a procedure, positioned her and, when she was turned toward the wall, handed the syringe to the medical student, indicating that she was to draw the spinal fluid. The student had seen the resident perform the procedure on the previous day. The resident then left the room. After several unsuccessful attempts, one medical student sought the resident who, on returning, said, "You've got to learn!"

COMMENT. There is no ethical problem in this case; it is an ethical outrage. No consideration was shown to the patient's feelings, appropriate informed consent was not obtained, supervision was inadequate, and easily arranged accommodations were not made. Students are often offended by being placed in such situations. As low persons in the medical school hierarchy, students may feel an ethical conflict and not know how, and to whom, to express their feelings.

Although the case described is an ethical outrage rather than an ethical problem, we must be aware that relatively inexperienced students perform many procedures in teaching hospitals, including blood drawing, intravenous insertions, lumbar punctures, paracenteses, thoracenteses, and occasional endotracheal intubations. Students often remark (in private) about their feelings concerning these procedures. They are eager to learn these skills and believe they must master these techniques to function effectively as physicians. Still, they are not sure how to approach the patient and how much disclosure is appropriate for the patient's informed consent, particularly for relatively innocuous, albeit discomforting, procedures, such as venipuncture.

Any senior person who orders a student to perform a clinical procedure assumes responsibility for the safe execution of the procedure and for its consequences. They should remain present when inexperienced students make their early attempts. Senior persons should invite students to express their discomfort or doubts about what they are asked to do.

Case II. A 74-year-old man with chronic obstructive pulmonary disease is admitted in mild respiratory failure with diffuse bronchospasm. His respiratory condition does not require insertion of a Swan-Ganz catheter for hemodynamic monitoring. Nevertheless, the chief resident suggests a catheter be placed; one of her reasons for this choice is to allow an inexperienced intern to practice this technical procedure.

COMMENT. Procedures involving any risk should be performed only for diagnostic or therapeutic purposes. Risky procedures should not be done exclusively or even partially for their teaching value. Thus, in Case II, the intern's need for additional practice should not affect the chief resident's clinical judgment. If the procedure is harmless, such as palpation or auscultation, or involves only minor inconvenience, such as asking a patient with ataxic gait to get up from a chair and walk across the room, or minor discomfort, such as extension and flexing of an arthritic limb, patients may be requested to allow the procedure. Noninvasive procedures, involving neither risk nor discomfort, such as auscultation or examination of pupils or skin, are permitted even on patients who are incapacitated without a decision-making capability.

Case III. A second-year medical student is being mentored by a surgeon in private practice. A 22-year-old woman has been prepared for an appendectomy and is now under anesthesia. The surgeon suggests that the student might do his first pelvic examination on the unconscious patient.

COMMENT. This is ethically unacceptable. The patient has not consented to this particularly intimate procedure and, even though unconscious, suffers an offense to her dignity. The student is embarrassed, both at doing the examination and at expressing his discomfort to his mentor. Medical schools should have careful guidelines on this subject and, if possible, arrange teaching experiences that are acceptable to students and to patients.

4.8.2 Teaching Procedures on the Newly Dead

Many teaching programs use recently dead patients to teach various nonmutilating procedures, including tracheal intubation, placement of central venous catheters, and pericardiocentesis. In one study, only 10% of the programs that used newly dead patients for teaching obtained either verbal or written consent from the patient's survivors. Proponents of training on the newly dead argue that it is beneficial to society, nonmutilating to the dead patient, and that no good alternatives are available. They further argue that consent need not be sought, because consent can be presumed for harmless procedures and because the grieving survivors should not be further troubled about something that is not harmful or mutilating to their deceased relative. It is our opinion that, although the newly dead may be used to teach some procedures, it is ethically and legally appropriate to seek consent from next of kin. This acknowledges that we recognize and respect the special status of the newly dead person; omitting consent is a violation of trust. Many families have religious or cultural beliefs that should be respected; also, secretive activities are offensive to many health professionals, including medical students, nurses, and society. Finally, a number of studies have shown that consent for procedures, such as endotracheal intubation, can frequently be obtained from family if approached in a sensitive and respectful manner.

4.9 OCCUPATIONAL MEDICINE

The occupational physician, the military physician, and the prison or police physician may encounter conflicts of interest. As physicians, they are obligated to serve those who come to them as patients; as employees, they have some obligations to their employers. Ethical problems may arise, particularly about confidentiality and disclosure.

Case I. The dialysis nurse described at Section 4.2.3 is examined by the hospital's Employee Health Service physician. This examination is required by hospital regulations. When the physician tells the nurse she is hepatitis B antigen–positive, she insists he not report her to the director of the dialysis unit.

COMMENT. The physician in this case has accepted responsibilities both to the institution and to particular patients. This dual relationship should be clear to the patient in this situation. The physician should report this patient. The dual relationship may not be clear in many situations where workers approach company physicians. It is imperative that the dual relationship be made clear whenever it is relevant and that its implications are spelled out for a patient-employee.

Case II. A worker in an industry using kepone visits the company physician about a persistent cough. The physician does a cursory physical and prescribes a cough medicine. It is company policy not to investigate symptoms of this sort too aggressively until they become demonstrably more serious. It is also policy not to suggest to worker-patients the potential for lung disease or to make employee health records available to them.

COMMENT. The company policy is manifestly unethical, because it causes persons who may be benefited by early diagnosis and treatment to be deprived of it through remediable ignorance. The physician who accepts such a policy clearly acts unethically, because duties to patients are disregarded without the patient's being made aware of the physician's dual role. The Code of Ethics of the American Society for Occupational Medicine requires physicians working in such settings to "avoid allowing medical judgment to be influenced by any conflict of interest" and "to accord highest priority to the health and safety of the individual in the work place." This implies that conflicts should be resolved in favor of individual patients, even if this is to the detriment of the company and the physician. Physicians accepting positions with dual responsibilities should be certain that their employers will allow them to abide by the ethical code.

The Code Of Ethics Of the American Society for Occupational Medicine. *Occup Med* 1976;8:Cover.

4.10 PUBLIC HEALTH

Public health is the science and practice of preventing disease and promoting health in populations. As a science, it depends largely on epidemiology and, as a practice, is largely performed by governmental organizations, such as the Centers for Disease Control and local health departments. The traditional objectives were the control of communicable disease, the safety of the water and food supply, and response to natural disasters. More recently, public health has turned to broad educational efforts to enhance the health of the public by warning of health risks, informing about healthy lifestyles, and encouraging preventive care, such as prenatal care. Since September 11, 2001, public health authorities have been called upon to deal with bioterrorism attacks and have been asked to develop plans to deal with biologic, chemical, and nuclear threats. Many of the ethical issues of public health are matters of policy and are beyond the scope of this book. However, public health intersects with clinical care at several points. The protection of the public from communicable diseases, for example, is occasionally in conflict with the medical duty of confidentiality. This is discussed at Section 4.2.3. One aspect of public health, the immunization of children, is a particular issue for pediatric ethics.

4.10.1 Immunization

Vaccination is a major public health measure and is important to the health of individual children. The long effort by pediatricians to institute mandatory or universal immunization is threatened by changes in public health law that permit persons whose religious beliefs oppose such procedures to refuse vaccination and by the growing perception of parents that vaccination has risks that could lead to serious and possibly uncompensated harm for their children. Although this is distressing, the basic principle must be recalled: Vaccination does put a child at some small risk of major harm to avoid a somewhat remote threat to the child's own health for the sake of contributing to the general safety of other children.

COMMENT. When immunization is compulsory by law, the pediatrician does not obtain "informed consent" (with its counterpart, "informed dissent") from the parents. Instead, full information is given about the necessity for immunization and its risks. If immunization is not compulsory, the pediatrician must respect the parents' wishes, although efforts to educate and persuade are suitable. If parents refuse immunization against a serious disease of epidemic proportions, legal authorization should be sought. Many states have religious exemption from immunization: Mississippi and West Virginia alone require all children to be immunized without exemption for religion. The problem of compensation for the harms caused by immunization is a matter of social policy. Pediatric medicine should work to ensure the establishment of an equitable system for compensation of those who are involuntarily exposed to risks for the public good.

4.11 ETHICS COMMITTEES

In the usual practice of medicine, important decisions are, and should be, made by the patient and physician together. Outside parties do not partake in those decisions unless invited to do so by the principal parties. The growing complexity of the ethical issues in clinical care has stimulated the development of ethics committees and of ethics consultation. Ethics committees are established in health care institutions as advisory groups on policy and sometimes on cases that involve ethical issues. It is their responsibility to be familiar with the literature and methods of the field of bioethics and to make available to those who seek their counsel the best informed opinions about issues. Many judicial opinions have endorsed the idea of ethics committees as a means of resolving disputes before the participants are forced to the courts.

Ethics committees differ from institutional review boards (IRBs), which focus on research involving human subjects and function in accordance with federal regulations. Ethics committees deal with policies and problems arising in the care of patients. The Joint Commission for Accreditation of Health Care Organizations (JCAHO) requires hospitals to have a mechanism to address ethical issues in patient care.

Joint Commission on American Hospital Organizations. *Accreditation Manual for Hospitals.* 1992.

The President's Commission for the Study of Ethical Problems in Medicine recommended that ethics committees have three functions: ed ucation, policy development, and case consultation. The Federal Patient Self-Determination Act of 1991, which required hospitals to ascertain whether newly admitted patients had advance directives and to provide education about their use, stimulated community educational activities, often undertaken by ethics committees and professional organizations.

Ethics committees develop institutional policies on matters such as DNAR or the management of patients in a persistent vegetative state. Another recent development is the use of dispute resolution techniques, such as informal negotiation or mediation as an alternative to litigation when conflicts arise between patients or families and physicians. Although the number of ethics committees has increased greatly in recent years, and very few US hospitals are without one, there are no rigorous studies to evaluate the effectiveness of these committees.

Evaluation of case consultation in clinical ethics. *J Clin Ethics* 1996;7(2).

An effective ethics committee has the following characteristics:

(a) Endorsement and support from the hospital administration and the medical and nursing staff. That support should include sufficient resources for the committee to function efficiently. The committee should be located clearly and appropriately in the institution's organizational chart, with designated lines of reporting.

(b) Members should be persons who are respected by their peers. The committee should also have members from outside the health care organization who represent a nonprofessional view of problems and may be able to speak for certain communities served by the organization. Members should meet regularly and keep records of their deliberations and of case consultations. Records should be maintained as confidential, according to the relevant laws.

(c) The committee should establish methods of informing the staff of its existence and role and the procedures whereby it is contacted. Educational functions, such as occasional grand rounds or noon conferences, should be sponsored.

(d) Members and potential members should be given the opportunity and support to pursue education in medical ethics. Many educational opportunities are now available throughout the country.

4.12 ETHICS CONSULTATION

Many hospitals and other health care institutions have employed ethics consultants or have authorized members of the ethics committee to engage in consultations on ethical problems arising in particular cases. Ethics consultation is modeled on the familiar practice of professional consultation: Certain persons who have training in the field of bioethics are available to practitioners, and occasionally to patients, to review the facts of a particular case and offer informed and prudent counsel suited to the case. Often the consultation service is one of the activities of the ethics committee.

The central goal of ethics consultation is to improve the process and outcome of care by identifying, analyzing, and working to resolve ethical problems encountered in individual cases. To achieve this goal, it is necessary to identify the issue that precipitated the consultation and to facilitate resolution through patient and staff education and the opportunity for informed and respectful discussion of the problem.

Competency for ethics consultation includes knowledge of bioethics, the relevant professional codes of ethics, and relevant health law. An ethics consultant should also have sufficient knowledge of medicine to assess the clinical situation, demonstrate skill at moral reasoning, and have the ability to build moral consensus in a group. A number of degree and certification programs provide education in bioethics. Ethics consultation has been evaluated in several retrospective studies that showed a reasonably high level of patient and physician satisfaction with the consultation.

COMMENT. The conclusions of the deliberations of ethics committees and of ethics consultation are usually reported to the attending physician. However, ethics consultants and ethics committees, risk managers, and legal counsel may collaborate with the attending physician and with patients and families to find informal solutions to ethical conflicts. For example, if physicians and parents disagree about the treatment plan for a severely and possibly terminally ill child, the dispute might be mediated by seeking an outside opinion from someone acceptable to physicians and parents. Even if physicians and parents fail to agree on everything, compromises might be achieved. If that fails, the parents have the option of transferring the child to a different institution. One general goal of an ethics program involving ethics committees and consultation is to identify and manage ethics conflicts by seeking solutions rather than provoking litigation. Those problems that cannot be resolved by informal procedures may require formal legal resolution.

RECOMMENDATION. We recommend that ethics committees and ethics consultants employ the method of analysis presented in this book.

Locator

This Locator is designed to provide the reader with rapid access to issues that are likely to be subjects of discussion in an ethical inquiry or in teaching clinical ethics. The entries indicate the major sections in which the issue is treated. Where there are more than a few citations, the principal section is marked in **boldface numbers**. Thus, if a discussion centers on whether a particular decision is in the best interest of an incapacitated patient, the reader looks up "Best Interest" and sees that the main treatment of this issue is found at **3.03**. Similarly, the main discussion of incapacity is found under "Decisional Capacity" at **2.2–2.2.3**. Ample internal references will also lead readers to further treatments of the issue.